Social Media and Pediatric Mental Health

Editors

ERIN L. BELFORT
PAUL E. WEIGLE

PEDIATRIC CLINICS
OF NORTH AMERICA

www.pediatric.theclinics.com

Consulting Editor
TINA L. CHENG

April 2025 • Volume 72 • Number 2

ELSEVIER

1600 John F. Kennedy Boulevard • Suite 1800 • Philadelphia, Pennsylvania, 19103-2899

http://www.theclinics.com

THE PEDIATRIC CLINICS OF NORTH AMERICA Volume 72, Number 2
April 2025 ISSN 0031-3955, ISBN-13: 978-0-443-29590-4

Editor: Kerry Holland
Developmental Editor: Anirban Mukherjee

The Pediatric Clinics of North America (ISSN 0031-3955) is published bimonthly by Elsevier Inc., 360 Park Avenue South, New York, NY 10010-1710. Months of issue are February, April, June, August, October, and December. Periodicals postage paid at New York, NY and additional mailing offices. Subscription prices are $299.00 per year (US individuals), $380.00 per year (Canadian individuals), $453.00 per year (international individuals), $100.00 per year (US students and residents), $100.00 per year (Canadian students and residents), and $165.00 per year (international residents and students). For institutional access pricing please contact Customer Service via the contact information below. To receive students/resident rare, orders must be accompanied by name of affiliated institution, date of term, and the signature of program/residency coordinator on institution letterhead. Orders will be billed at individual rate until proof of status is received. Foreign air speed delivery is included in all Clinics subscription prices. All prices are subject to change without notice. Orders, claims, and journal inquiries: Please visit our Support Hub page https://service.elsevier.com for assistance.

Reprints. For copies of 100 or more, of articles in this publication, please contact the Commercial Reprints Department, Elsevier Inc., 360 Park Avenue South, New York, NY 10010-1710. Tel.: 212-633-3874; Fax: 212-633-3820; E-mail: reprints@elsevier.com.

The Pediatric Clinics of North America is also published in Spanish by McGraw-Hill Inter-americana Editores S.A., Mexico City, Mexico; in Portuguese by Riechmann and Affonso Editores, Rua Comandante Coelho 1085, CEP 21250, Rio de Janeiro, Brazil; and in Greek by Althayia SA, Athens, Greece.

The Pediatric Clinics of North America is covered in MEDLINE/PubMed (Index Medicus), Excerpta Medica, Current Contents, Current Contents/Clinical Medicine, Science Citation Index, ASCA, ISI/BIOMED, and BIOSIS.

PROGRAM OBJECTIVE

The goal of the *Pediatric Clinics of North America* is to keep practicing physicians and residents up to date with current clinical practice in pediatrics by providing timely articles reviewing the state-of-the-art in patient care.

TARGET AUDIENCE

All practicing pediatricians, physicians, and healthcare professionals who provide patient care to pediatric patients.

LEARNING OBJECTIVES

Upon completion of this activity, participants will be able to:

1. Review strategies clinicians use when evaluating youth who use social media to self diagnose.
2. Discuss the role of social media and its impact on adolescent self-esteem.
3. Recognize the upsurge in youth screen time and social media usage coincides with increasing mental health concerns.

ACCREDITATIONS

Physician Credit

The Elsevier Office of Continuing Medical Education (EOCME) is accredited by the Accreditation Council for Continuing Medical Education (ACCME) to provide continuing medical education for physicians.

The EOCME designates this journal-based activity for a maximum of 14 *AMA PRA Category 1 Credit*(s)™. Physicians should claim only the credit commensurate with the extent of their participation in the activity.

All other healthcare professionals requesting continuing education credit for this journal-based activity will be issued a certificate of participation.

ABP Maintenance of Certification Credit

Successful completion of this CME activity, which includes participation in the activity and individual assessment of and feedback to the learner, enables the learner to earn up to 14 MOC points in the American Board of Pediatrics' (ABP) Maintenance of Certification (MOC) program. It is the CME activity provider's responsibility to submit learner completion information to ACCME for the purpose of granting ABP MOC credit.

DISCLOSURE OF RELEVANT FINANCIAL RELATIONSHIPS

The EOCME assesses conflict of interest with its instructors, faculty, planners, and other individuals who are in a position to control the content of CME activities. All relevant conflicts of interest that are identified are thoroughly vetted by EOCME for fair balance, scientific objectivity, and patient care recommendations. EOCME is committed to providing its learners with CME activities that promote improvements or quality in healthcare and not a specific proprietary business or a commercial interest.

The authors and editors listed below have identified no financial relationships or relationships to products or devices they have with ineligible companies related to the content of this CME activity:
Seeba Anam, MD; Merlin Ariefdjohan, PhD, MPH; Sahar Ashraf, MD; Jenni Auqui, BA; Erin Belfort, MD; Casey Berson, MD; Zhamilya Bilyalova; Christopher Chamanadjian, MD; Jeremy Chapman, MD; Linda Charmaraman, PhD; Ailyn D. Diaz, MD; Elizabeth K. Englander, PhD; Sandra Fritsch, MD, MSEd, DFAACAP; Meredith Gansner, MD; Roslyn L. Gerwin, DO; Fadi J. Hamati, MD; Jane Harness, DO; Lauren E. Hartstein, PhD; Horacio Hojman, MD, MBA; Zainub Javed, MD; Kristopher Kaliebe, MD; Dale Aaron Peeples, MD; Dana Reid, DO; Bushra Rizwan, MD; Kaushal Shah, MD, MPH; Ashvin Sood, MD; Clifford Sussman, MD, PLLC; Daniel J. Suto, BS, MD; Jack L. Turban, MD; Carol Vidal, MD, PhD; Paul Weigle, MD; Jennifer L. Yen, MD, FAACAP

The authors and editors listed below have identified financial relationships or relationships to products or devices they have with ineligible companies related to the content of this CME activity:
T. Atilla Ceranoglu, MD: *Researcher*: Niraxx, Inc.

Lauren Hale, PhD: *Consultant*: Idorsia Pharmaceuticals Ltd.

The planning committee and staff listed below have identified no financial relationships or relationships to products or devices they have with ineligible companies related to the content of this CME activity:
Kerry Holland; Shyamala Kavikumaran; Michelle Littlejohn; Patrick J. Manley; Anirban Mukherjee

UNAPPROVED/OFF-LABEL USE DISCLOSURE

The EOCME requires CME faculty to disclose to the participants:

1. When products or procedures being discussed are off-label, unlabelled, experimental, and/or investigational (not US Food and Drug Administration [FDA] approved); and
2. Any limitations on the information presented, such as data that are preliminary or that represent ongoing research, interim analyses, and/or unsupported opinions. Faculty may discuss information about pharmaceutical agents that is outside of FDA-approved labelling. This information is intended solely for CME and is not intended to promote off-label use of these medications. If you have any questions, contact the medical affairs department of the manufacturer for the most recent prescribing information.

TO ENROLL

To enroll in the *Pediatric Clinics of North America* Continuing Medical Education program, call customer service at 1-800-654-2452 or sign up online at https://www.pediatric.theclinics.com/cme/home. The CME program is available to subscribers for an additional annual fee of USD 313.00.

METHOD OF PARTICIPATION

In order to claim credit, participants must complete the following:

1. Complete enrolment as indicated above.
2. Read the activity.
3. Complete the CME Test and Evaluation. Participants must achieve a score of 70% on the test. All CME Tests and Evaluations must be completed online.

In order to claim MOC points, participants must complete the following:

1. Complete steps listed above for claiming CME credit
2. Provide your specialty board ID#, birth date (MM/DD), and attestation.
3. Online MOC submission is only available for the American Board of pediatrics' (ABP) Maintenance of Certification (MOC) program

CME INQUIRIES/SPECIAL NEEDS

For all CME inquiries or special needs, please contact elsevierCME@elsevier.com.

Contributors

CONSULTING EDITOR

TINA L. CHENG, MD, MPH
BK Rachford Professor and Chair of Pediatrics, University of Cincinnati, Director, Cincinnati Children's Research Foundation, Chief Medical Officer, Cincinnati Children's Hospital Medical Center, Cincinnati, Ohio

EDITORS

ERIN L. BELFORT, MD
Child and Adolescent Psychiatry Fellowship Training Director, Department of Psychiatry, Maine Medical Center, Portland, Maine, Associate Professor of Psychiatry, Tufts University School of Medicine, Boston, MA, USA

PAUL E. WEIGLE, MD
Child and Adolescent Psychiatrist, Associate Medical Director, Outpatient Services, Natchaug Hospital, Hartford Healthcare, Mansfield Center, Mansfield, Associate Professor, Department of Psychiatry, University of Connecticut School of Medicine, Farmington, Connecticut, USA

AUTHORS

SEEBA ANAM, MD
Associate Professor, Department of Psychiatry and Behavioral Neuroscience, University of Chicago, Chicago, Illinois, USA

MERLIN ARIEFDJOHAN, PhD, MPH
Assistant Professor, Department of Psychiatry, University of Colorado Anschutz Medical Campus, Aurora, Colorado, USA

SAHAR ASHRAF, MD
Child and Adolescent Psychiatry Fellow, Department of Psychiatry, Texas Tech University Health Science Center, Midland, Texas, USA

JENNI QUICHIMBO AUQUI, BA
Research Intern, Youth, Media & Wellbeing Research Lab, Wellesley Centers for Women, Wellesley College, Wellesley, Massachusetts, USA

ERIN L. BELFORT, MD
Child and Adolescent Psychiatry Fellowship Training Director, Department of Psychiatry, Maine Medical Center, Portland, Maine, Associate Professor of Psychiatry, Tufts University School of Medicine, Boston, MA, USA

CASEY BERSON, MD
Child Psychiatrist, Prisma Health, Greer, South Carolina, USA

ZHAMILYA BILYALOVA
Research Intern, Youth, Media & Wellbeing Research Lab, Wellesley Centers for Women, Wellesley College, Wellesley, Massachusetts, USA

TOLGA ATILLA CERANOGLU, MD
Assistant Professor, Department of Psychiatry, Harvard Medical School, Boston, Massachusetts, USA

CHRISTOPHER CHAMANADJIAN, MD
Child and Adolescent Psychiatry Fellow, Department of Psychiatry, Arrowhead Regional Medical Center, California, USA

JEREMY A. CHAPMAN, MD
Medical Director of Child Psychiatry, Department of Psychiatry, SSM Health Treffert Center and Treffert Studios, Fond du Lac, Wisconsin, USA

LINDA CHARMARAMAN, PhD
Senior Research Scientist, Youth, Media & Wellbeing Research Lab, Wellesley Centers for Women, Wellesley College, Wellesley, Massachusetts, USA

AILYN D. DIAZ, MD
Associate Professor, Division of Child and Adolescent Psychiatry, Department of Psychiatry and Behavioral Health, Pennsylvania State University College of Medicine, Hershey, Pennsylvania, USA

ELIZABETH K. ENGLANDER, PhD
Executive Director, Massachusetts Aggression Reduction Center, Bridgewater State University, Bridgewater, Massachusetts, USA

SANDRA FRITSCH, MD, MSEd, DFAACAP
Professor, Department of Psychiatry, University of Colorado Anschutz Medical Campus, Medical Director, Pediatric Mental Health Institute, Children's Hospital Colorado, Anschutz Medical Campus, Aurora, Colorado

MEREDITH GANSNER, MD
Child Psychiatrist, Department of Psychiatry, Boston Children's Hospital, Boston, Massachusetts, USA

ROSLYN L. GERWIN, DO
Assistant Clinical Professor of Psychiatry, Tufts University School of Medicine, Boston, Massachusetts, USA; Director, Department of Child and Adolescent Psychiatry, Pediatric Psychiatry Consultation Service, Barbara Bush Children's Hospital, Maine Medical Center, Portland, Maine, USA

LAUREN HALE, PhD
Professor, Program in Public Health, Department of Family, Population, and Preventive Medicine, Renaissance School of Medicine, Stony Brook University, Stony Brook, New York, USA

FADI J. HAMATI, MD
Psychiatry Resident Physician, Department of Psychiatry, Northwestern Memorial Hospital, Chicago, Illinois, USA

JANE HARNESS, DO
Clinical Assistant Professor, Department of Psychiatry, University of Michigan, Ann Arbor, Michigan, USA

LAUREN E. HARTSTEIN, PhD
Postdoctoral Fellow, Department of Integrative Physiology, University of Colorado Boulder, Boulder, Colorado, USA

HORACIO HOJMAN, MD, MBA
Clinical Professor, Department of Psychiatry and Human Behavior, Alpert Medical School, Brown University, Providence, Rhode Island, USA

ZAINUB JAVED, MD
PGY-3 Resident Physician, Department of Psychiatry , Prisma Health/University of South Carolina School of Medicine, Greenville, Greer, SC, USA

KRISTOPHER KALIEBE, MD
Professor, Department of Psychiatry and Behavioral Neurosciences, University of South Florida, Tampa, Florida, USA

DALE AARON PEEPLES, MD
Associate Professor, Department of Psychiatry, Medical College of Georgia at Augusta University, Augusta, Georgia, USA

DANA REID, DO
Child, Adolescent and Adult Psychiatrist, Private Practice, Alpharetta, Georgia, USA

BUSHRA RIZWAN, MD
Assistant Professor, Division of Child and Adolescent Psychiatry, Department of Psychiatry and Behavioral Sciences, Johns Hopkins Hospital, Attending Psychiatrist, Department of Developmental Behavioral Health, Kennedy Krieger Institute, Baltimore, Maryland, USA

KAUSHAL SHAH, MD, MPH
Psychiatric Residency, Department of Psychiatry, Wake Forest University, Winston-Salem, North Carolina, USA

ASHVIN SOOD, MD
Adult, Child and Adolescent Psychiatrist, Department of Psychiatry, SSM Health Treffert Center and Treffert Studios, Fond du Lac, Wisconsin, USA

CLIFFORD SUSSMAN, MD, PLLC
Clinical Instructor and Volunteer Clinical Faculty, Department of Psychiatry and Behavioral Health, George Washington University Medical School, Washington, DC, USA

DANIEL J. SUTO, BS, MD
Resident, Department of Emergency Medicine, University of California, San Francisco, Zuckerberg San Francisco General Hospital, San Francisco, California, USA

JACK L. TURBAN, MD
Assistant Professor of Child and Adolescent Psychiatry, Department of Psychiatry, University of California, San Francisco, San Francisco, California, USA

CAROL VIDAL, MD, PhD
Assistant Professor, Department of Psychiatry and Behavioral Sciences, Johns Hopkins University School of Medicine, Baltimore, Maryland, USA

PAUL E. WEIGLE, MD
Child and Adolescent Psychiatrist, Associate Medical Director, Outpatient Services, Natchaug Hospital, Hartford Healthcare, Mansfield Center, Mansfield; Associate

Professor, Department of Psychiatry, University of Connecticut School of Medicine, Farmington, Connecticut, USA

JENNIFER L. YEN, MD, FAACAP
Clinical Assistant Professor, Department of Psychiatry and Behavioral Sciences, Baylor College of Medicine; Child and Adolescent Psychiatrist, The Harris Center for Mental Health and IDD, Houston, Texas, USA

Contents

media is widely used by youth, with widespread effects, including the potential to influence the development of disordered eating. Higher risk youth can be vulnerable to advertising, body image comparisons, and predatory online eating disorder communities.

As in traditional media, the depiction of ideas and behaviors on social media can influence viewers to adopt them. Social media may be particularly influential because the platforms are highly engaging, reach a vast audience, and personalize user experience to feature content most likely to affect the individual user. Numerous high-risk adolescent behaviors have been linked to viewing related social media content, but the extent to which they are the cause of and caused by content exposure remains unknown. Pediatric providers are advised to adopt standardized approaches to the prevention and management of social media contagion in clinical practice.

Sexting (sending a nude picture of oneself to another person) is a common, but not universal, behavior between adolescents. This article presents research on 2252 18 year old individuals studied between 2020 and 2022. Around 52% sent a sext to a peer. Approximately 70% experienced negative or positive pressure from peers or self-pressure. Approximately 77% of negative-pressured sexters reported challenges with anxiety, compared to 58% of positive-pressured sexters and 41% of non-sexters. This paper also presents typical and atypical sexting cases and notes clinical implications of the research findings.

Medical professionals should be mindful of social media's impact on attention, especially for youth who already has limited ability to focus due to neurocognitive difficulties or emotional disorders. Digital distractions often interfere with academic performance. Social media interactions displace other means for youth to learn about the world and contribute to the spread of misinformation. Attentional literacy is a method of combating digital distraction and misinformation by promoting an intentional application of focus. Addressing information overload and misinformation requires individuals and institutions to actively manage attentional resources and employ thoughtful content analysis.

Social media (SM) use has become ubiquitous in adolescent life, raising concerns about its impact on their mental health. While research has identified links between excessive SM use and negative mental health outcomes, the relationship remains complex. The authors propose a novel function-based framework and algorithm that aids clinicians in evaluating SM use, independent of platform-specific knowledge. By eliciting the patterns of engagement and social interactions, the proposed framework aims to identify associated risk and resilience factors, thereby informing screening, assessment, and intervention strategies for adolescents in this ever-growing digital landscape.

While social media has been a catalyst for mental health awareness, the unregulated dissemination of information by influencers lacking mental health expertise, perpetuates misinformation. Youth commonly self-diagnose mental health conditions based on social media content, often inaccurately, risking misidentification and inappropriate treatment. Psychiatric contagion, the process by which psychiatric symptoms spread among individuals in close contact, can occur via social media. The authors explore how these issues present in clinical practice, and some intervention strategies for clinicians. They offer recommendations for parents, teachers, social media companies, and clinicians.

Sexual and gender development are key components of adolescence. As social media becomes increasingly ingrained in youth culture, it is essential to understand its impact on these developmental pathways. Social media provides a novel avenue for adolescents to explore identity, sexuality, and intimacy—as well as newfound autonomy and risk taking. Adolescents typically use social media for age-appropriate interactions and many find mental health benefits, alongside potential risks to mental and physical health. Clinicians should use a nonjudgmental tone to inquire about adolescent online behaviors and to counsel patients on safe and developmentally appropriate identity and relationship development.

With the advent of smartphones and the popularization of social media sites at the beginning of the twenty-first century, children and adolescents have been exposed to a world of virtual interactions in social networking sites that are designed to increase engagement of the user for profit. In this article, we review the epidemiology of use of social media, its addictive features, and potential negative consequences of problematic use, and the research on current interventions known to reduce use. We also give recommendations spanning from the policy to the individual level for children to build a healthier relationship with these sites.

In this article, we discuss a broad overview of the relationship between social media and youth mental health, including the legal and historical context of social media, role and involvement of caregivers, and strategies for modulation of usage. Additionally, we highlight the unique risk and protective factors of social media use for youth from marginalized groups, including exposure to racism and discrimination. We recommend social media companies avoid existing precedents regarding preferential censorship that has disadvantaged and caused harm to historically, persistently, or systematically marginalized groups.

Merlin Ariefdjohan, Dana Reid, and Sandra Fritsch

The upsurge in youth screen time and social media usage parallels growing mental health concerns. While causality remains unproven, many studies associate screen and social media use as anxiety risk factors. Social media can benefit some youth in forming connections and shaping identity, but it may also trigger or exacerbate anxiety, emphasizing the need for balanced and mindful use. This article reviews existing literature on the potential risks and benefits of screen and social media use on youth anxiety, and proposes strategies for managing mental and digital health challenges attributed by the rapidly evolving landscape of youth engagement with technology.

Jennifer L. Yen and Christopher Chamanadjian

With the rapid progress of technology and the Internet, the popularity of social media among youth as a preferred form of communication has grown exponentially. In addition to many of the challenges youth face in real life, much of their identity and development now occurs in online spaces as well. Traditional bullying has evolved into cyberbullying, which has been labeled a public health issue. Though both forms of bullying share similar characteristics, risk factors, and potential consequences, research on cyberbullying has revealed the need for new and novel interventions aimed at mitigating its negative impact on youth mental health.

PEDIATRIC CLINICS OF NORTH AMERICA

Foreword

Growing Up Online: The Impact of Social Media

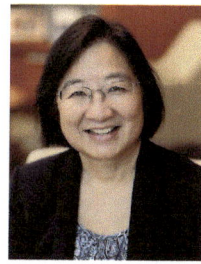

Tina L. Cheng, MD, MPH
Consulting Editor

What can we say about social media? We love it; we hate it. It's good; it's bad. Regardless, it is here to stay. Children and adolescents have grown up with social media, and 95% of US teenagers have a smartphone. But how does social media affect the health of children and adolescents?

The US Surgeon General[1] issued an advisory urging action to protect children online, and the American Psychological Association[2] issued its first-ever health advisory on social media use in adolescence. Two current bills supported by the American Academy of Pediatrics include the Kids Online Safety Act (KOSA) and the Children and Teens' Online Privacy Protection Act (COPPA 2.0). Recently, the Prime Minister of Australia proposed legislation to ban social media for anyone under 16 years of age. This issue of *Pediatric Clinics of North America* is timely in reviewing the impact of social media specifically on mental health. It also addresses how to discuss social media in clinical encounters.

The American Psychological Association[2] has defined social media as "technologically-based applications, platforms, or communication systems using online architecture that promotes asynchronous, unilateral, permanent, public, continually-accessible, social cue-restricted, quantifiable, visually-based, or algorithmic-based social interactions." It is hard to keep up with the different forms of social media, and young people are often educating me!

So, what is the impact on health? Earlier this year, the National Academy of Science, Engineering, and Medicine[3] released a report on "Social Media and Adolescent Health" reviewing the research on the impact of social media on the health and well-being of adolescents. They concluded that there was a "lack of robust evidence on the relationship between social media use and health outcomes" and proposed a

Pediatr Clin N Am 72 (2025) xv–xvi
https://doi.org/10.1016/j.pcl.2024.11.001
0031-3955/25/© 2024 Published by Elsevier Inc.

research agenda and recommendations to protect young people. Lack of evidence doesn't mean there isn't an impact on health but that more research is needed.

This issue of *Pediatric Clinics of North America* helps us stay informed. As social media platforms and research evolve, it is critical for us to keep up and discuss social media use with patients and families.

Tina L. Cheng, MD, MPH
Cincinnati Children's Hospital Medical Center
University of Cincinnati
Cincinnati Children's Research Foundation
3333 Burnet Avenue, MLC 3016
Cincinnati, OH 45229-3026, USA

E-mail address:
Tina.cheng@cchmc.org

REFERENCES

1. Social Media and Youth Mental Health. The U.S. Surgeon General's Advisory. 2023. Available at: https://www.hhs.gov/sites/default/files/sg-youth-mental-health-social-media-advisory.pdf. Accessed November 10, 2024.
2. American Psychological Association. Health advisory on social media use in adolescence. 2023. Available at: https://www.apa.org/topics/social-media-internet/health-advisory-adolescent-social-media-use. Accessed November 10, 2024.
3. National Academies of Sciences, Engineering, and Medicine. Social media and adolescent health. Washington, DC: The National Academies Press; 2024. Available at: https://www.nationalacademies.org/our-work/assessment-of-the-impact-of-social-media-on-the-health-and-wellbeing-of-adolescents-and-children. Accessed November 10, 2024.

Preface

Online and in Crisis: When Social Media Impacts Mental Health

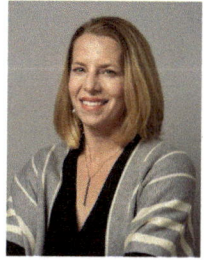 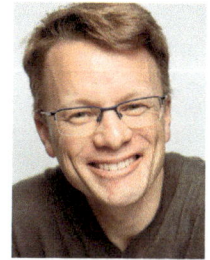

Erin L. Belfort, MD   Paul E. Weigle, MD
Editors

You open the exam room door to find Maya, age 15, on the exam table. You've cared for Maya and her siblings for many years, and you are seeing her for a well-child check. You notice that Maya scored highly on the PHQ-9 scale completed for the visit. Maya discloses that she's been feeling stressed about school and conflict with friends. She reports that she's "up and down" but often feeling irritated and annoyed, particularly when her mother tells her to do chores or get off her phone. During your exam, you notice some cuts on her upper arms in various stages of healing. You inquire about the cuts, and she admits to cutting herself with a razor blade for the last six months and hiding it from her mother. She often cannot sleep at night, so has been watching self-injury videos on her phone in her bedroom and chats with online gamer friends via Discord. It feels good to know that other kids are depressed, and they empathize and discuss how cutting can relieve distress. "They all think I am bipolar."

You glance at your watch, knowing that your time with Maya is short and that there are patients waiting to see you. You have several critical questions. Does Maya have major depression or bipolar disorder, or is something else going on? Are there imminent safety concerns? What unspoken stressors are at play, such as trauma or family conflict? What is the role of social media in encouraging Maya's self-injurious behavior, and how does it affect her sleep? Are online friendships helping her cope or making things worse? How should you advise Maya and her mother?

Maya's situation represents an increasingly common clinical scenario. As social media plays an increasingly important role in the everyday lives of youth, social media habits and experiences have greater consequences for mental health and well-being. The 2023 US Surgeon General Advisory about the effects of youth social media use on their mental health has only reinforced what pediatricians are seeing every day.

Pediatr Clin N Am 72 (2025) xvii–xviii
https://doi.org/10.1016/j.pcl.2024.10.002
0031-3955/25/© 2024 Published by Elsevier Inc.

pediatric.theclinics.com

However, pediatricians typically know less about social media than their young patients, and teasing out its impacts on any given patient can seem a labyrinthine task.

This issue of *Pediatric Clinics of North America* explores the nuanced relationship between social media and the mental health of youth. We describe how social media impacts mental health through important mediators, such as sleep, self-image, and emerging social and sexual identity and expression. We then turn to novel dilemmas created by clinical manifestations of social media use: sexting, cyberbullying, self-diagnosis, and digital distraction, and how best to assess and address them. We consider media's interaction with the common psychiatric conditions of depression, anxiety, and eating disorders. We describe social media contagion of mental health problems and problematic (eg, addictive) social media use. Finally, we detail how assessment of social media habits and experiences can be incorporated into a pediatric exam in order to screen for, evaluate, and address related influences on mental health.

Social media has transformed childhood and adolescence, and pediatricians must keep up. By exploring how social media and mental health interact, we can best understand our patients and guide them toward happier and healthier lives, online and off.

DISCLOSURE

The authors have no commercial or financial conflicts of interest.

Erin L. Belfort, MD
Department of Psychiatry
Maine Medical Center
22 Bramhall Street
Portland, ME 04102, USA

Tufts University School of Medicine
Boston, MA, USA

Paul E. Weigle, MD
Department of Psychiatry
University of Connecticut
School of Medicine
200 Academic Way
Farmington, CT 06032, USA

E-mail addresses:
Erin.Belfort@MaineHealth.org (E.L. Belfort)
paul.weigle@hhchealth.org (P.E. Weigle)

Social Media and Sleep Health

Lauren Hale, PhD[a],*, Lauren E. Hartstein, PhD[b],
Tolga Atilla Ceranoglu, MD[c]

KEYWORDS

• Social media • Sleep health • Pediatric populations • Mental health

KEY POINTS

• Social media, especially in the evening and during the night, interferes with pediatric sleep health.
• Proposed mechanisms for these effects include: activity displacement, arousal from content, alerting effects of light, and disruptions from noises and vibrations at night.
• Effective scalable interventions should be developed and evaluated.
• Clinicians and parents should work with youth to reduce the negative effects of social media use on sleep health.

INTRODUCTION

Social media permeates the daily lives of many children and adolescents.[1,2] Youth frequently use smartphones and other mobile devices during the evening and nighttime hours, interfering with sleep health. In this article, we provide current evidence on the importance of sleep health among pediatric populations, and what recent research reveals about the relationship between social media use and sleep. We discuss limitations of the existing research and conclude with recommendations for youth, families, and clinicians to help mitigate the possible adverse effects of social media use on sleep.

Funding: L. Hale is partially supported by grants from NICHD (R01 HD073352 and R21 HD097491) and the Della Pietra Family Foundation. L.E. Hartstein receives research support from NICHD (F32 HD103390).
a Program in Public Health, Department of Family, Population, and Preventive Medicine, Renaissance School of Medicine, Stony Brook University, Stony Brook, NY 11768-8338, USA;
b Department of Integrative Physiology, University of Colorado Boulder, Boulder, CO, USA;
c Department of Psychiatry, Harvard Medical School, Boston, MA, USA
* Corresponding author.
E-mail address: lauren.hale@stonybrook.edu

PEDIATRIC SLEEP HEALTH AFFECTS MENTAL HEALTH AND OTHER DEVELOPMENTAL OUTCOMES

Sleep serves numerous physiologic functions among pediatric populations, including regulation and maintenance of cardiovascular, metabolic, immune, cognitive, behavioral, and mental health.[3] Decades of research indicate that sufficient restorative sleep is an essential part of healthy development, impacting cognitive (executive functioning and academic performance),[4,5] emotional (emotional regulation, internalizing, and externalizing behaviors),[4,6–8] and physical outcomes (growth trajectories, obesity, and other cardiovascular risk factors)[7–10] from birth to adolescence.[11] Expert consensus panels recommend that school-aged children require between 9 and 12 h of sleep per night and that teenagers require 8 to 10 h per night for optimal development.[12,13] However, recent surveys reveal that the average amount of sleep among adolescents have declined over the last 2 decades. In the United States (US), 75% of youth report they sleep less than 8 h on school nights.[14,15] In Europe, less than half of the children and adolescents meet sleep recommendations.[16,17] Several characteristics of digital media access among youth consistently correlate with changes in sleep parameters, including bedtime, sleep onset, and total sleep duration. Location, duration, and timing of access to digital media have the strongest impact with sleep problems. Effective clinical interventions for sleep problems in youth must address maladaptive patterns of media use.[18–23]

Current State of Research on Social Media and Pediatric Sleep Health

Multiple systematic literature reviews document a widespread and consistent positive association between greater digital media use and poor sleep health among youth, ranging from pre-school-aged children through adolescents. These studies demonstrate that more digital media use is associated with delayed bedtimes, longer sleep-onset latency, shorter total sleep time, and more daytime sleepiness among children and adolescents.[24–30] The association between the presence of digital media in children's bedrooms and increased prevalence of sleep problems is a strong, consistent finding.[31–34]

When looking specifically at the association between social media and sleep health, similar patterns emerge. More interactive types of digital media (eg, social media, messaging) and smartphones that interrupt nighttime sleep are associated with a range of negative sleep outcomes including later bedtimes, longer sleep onset latency, shorter sleep duration, and poorer sleep quality.[24,27,35–37] For example, using the data from nearly 12,000 adolescents (13–15 year olds) in the Millennium Cohort Study, Scott and colleagues[37] shows a dose-response relationship between duration of social media use and later sleep onset, later wake times, and insomnia symptoms. In contrast, more passive types of media use (eg, streaming video content and watching television) show less consistent associations with sleep health outcomes.[24,28]

Social Media Before Bed and During the Night Adversely Affects Sleep

Both timing of the exposure and content of social media relate to sleep health. Bedtime and nighttime use of screens may have an even greater impact on poor sleep outcomes.[29,38,39] A 2016 meta-analysis including 20 cross-sectional studies from greater than 125,000 children found bedtime mobile phone use was associated with higher rates of insufficient sleep duration (odds ration[OR] = 2.17, 95% confidence interval [CI] 1.42–3.32), poor sleep quality (OR = 1.46, 95% CI 1.14–1.88), and excessive daytime sleepiness (OR = 2.72, 95% CI, 1.32–5.61).[29] In contrast to pre-sleep and nighttime screen use, studies of screen use (or social media specifically) during the day and/or further from bedtime have more inconsistent effects.[24] Several intervention studies demonstrate limiting screen use in the hours before bed significantly improves sleep health.[40,41] For example, Perrault and colleagues[40] found that limiting screen time after 9:00 PM in a sample of 569 adolescents resulted in earlier bedtimes and greater sleep duration. Bartel and colleagues, showed similar benefits for 63 adolescents asked to put their phones away in the hour before bed.[41] Screen media restrictions are challenging for parents to enforce and some intervention studies restricting screen use failed to show significant improvements in sleep health.[42,43]

Proposed Mechanisms that Explain the Link Between Social Media and Sleep Health

The association between screen-based digital media use and sleep health outcomes is often attributed to 4 plausible pathways, briefly described as follows, with a focus on social media effects on sleep.

Activity displacement

The first proposed mechanism is about time use—specifically that time spent on social media displaces sleep by delaying both the times youth get into bed and when they shut their eyes (which may distinct if the phone is brought into bed), thus shortening overall sleep duration. The time spent using social media would otherwise be used for preparing for sleep (eg, reading from a book, getting ready for the next morning) or actually sleeping.[25] Similarly, social media and other screen use may displace other health behaviors beneficial for sleep, such as daytime exposure to outdoor light and physical activity. Support for the activity displacement hypothesis is provided by long shut-eye latency periods in which adolescents get in bed, but delay shutting their eyes for a long time in order to engage with screen media.[44,45]

Psychologic stimulation from social media content

The second proposed pathway involves content-related stimulation that increases alertness and therefore impairs the ability to fall asleep. This could include arousal from social media or messaging,[25,46] with related experiences of social comparison, as well as online conflict and aggression, both of which may lead to negative thoughts, emotions, and memories.[38,47] Van der Schurr shows that social media stress is associated with longer sleep latency and daytime sleepiness.[46] Research by Vernon and colleagues[48,49] demonstrates a positive association between problematic social media use and sleep disruptions. Independent of psychologic arousal, physiologic arousal associated with video gaming has been shown to correlate with changes to sleep architecture by delaying sleep onset, shortening sleep duration, and reducing sleep efficiency.[18,50–52]

Effects of nighttime light exposure on circadian physiology and alertness

The light emitted by screens, particularly when it contains short-wavelength blue light,[53] disrupt sleep by suppressing release of the sleep-promoting hormone melatonin, delaying the timing of the circadian clock, and decreasing nighttime sleepiness.[39,54–56] These effects may be particularly strong in children, who have both clearer lenses and larger pupils than adults, allowing more light into the eye to stimulate the retina.[57–60] However, studies using light-adjusting software that alters the spectrum light emitted by screen devices in order to be less stimulating to the circadian system have reported little to no effects on sleep outcomes or melatonin secretion.[61–63] In an experimental study with young adults, participants viewed either their own or a mock Facebook page on a tablet with either blue-filtered or full wavelength light.[64] The combination of blue-filtered light and the "low arousal" non-personal account resulted in significantly better subjective sleep quality than either manipulation alone, suggesting that media interventions, which address multiple underlying pathways to sleep health, are more likely successful.

Nighttime sleep disruption

Sleep may be disrupted by noises and vibrations from cell phone notifications, as well as unease related to fear of missing out (FOMO) on social interactions. A 2019 report indicated that more than one-third of teens use their phones during the night for activities other than checking the time, most frequently because they received a notification (54%) or to check social media (51%).[65] In a study of undergraduate students, nighttime cell phone notifications significantly predicted self-reported global sleep problems and sleep disruptions, while a greater compulsion to check notifications at night predicted poorer sleep quality.[66] FOMO can contribute to short sleep duration in adolescence by increasing both nighttime social media use and pre-sleep cognitive arousal,[67] leading to delayed bedtimes and a longer time to fall asleep.

LIMITATIONS

Although cross-sectional, observational research studies consistently demonstrate a strong association between increased social media use and poor sleep health, experimental studies establishing a causal relationship are lacking. The majority of studies to date employ either self- or parent-report measures of screen use and sleep, which may be subject to bias.[68–71] Objective measures of social media use (eg, passive sensing) and sleep duration/timing (eg, actigraphy, polysomnography) may more accurately assess how patterns and characteristics of social media use (timing, duration, frequency, and content) affect sleep. Finally, further research is needed to develop feasible, sustainable, and effective interventions to help youth regulate their social media use in order to promote sleep health, particularly in light of findings that social media use can have both positive and negative impacts on adolescents' well-being.[72] A 2017 focus group of adolescents and young adults (aged 16–25 years) found that most wished to improve their sleep behavior, but had experienced limited success due in part to difficulty curtailing technology and social media use.[73] A systematic review and meta-analysis examining the efficacy of interventions to reduce children's screen use and enhance sleep suggests that modest declines in media use and related improvements in sleep health can be achieved.[74] Across 11 studies which included children aged 2 to 13 years, interventions resulted in an average reduction in screen use of 33 min per day and average sleep duration increased by 11 min per day. Limitations of the analysis include the large variability across the intervention strategies and type of media use targeted (eg, TV, video games, and overall screen use), as well as the primary focus of several interventions on outcomes other than media reduction and sleep (eg, weight-related behaviors). The association between the presence of digital media in children's bedrooms and increased prevalence of sleep problems is a strong, consistent finding.[31–34]

CLINICAL IMPLICATIONS AND RECOMMENDATIONS FOR YOUTH, FAMILIES, AND CLINICIANS

Recommendations

We offer the following public-facing recommendations to youth, families, teachers, coaches, clinicians, and policy makers. These are based on the most recent research and build upon our prior recommendations[75] and those endorsed by the American Academy of Pediatrics (AAP).[1]

- Prioritize sleep: Discussions with children regarding the importance of sleep and expectations for health sleep should be conducted in multiple settings (eg, homes, classrooms, after-school activities, and doctor visits).
- Maintain bedtime routines, which avoid disruptive digital media use and focus on calming activities.
- Remove all digital media from youths' bedrooms: smartphones, televisions, video games, computers, and tablets.
- To prevent children from surreptitiously using screen media at night, consider disconnecting or disabling Wi-Fi router at bedtime, charging children's tablets and phones in the parents' bedroom, and setting device parental controls to disallow nighttime use.
- For youth with sleep problems, ensure the steps above are observed before using sleep medication.

CLINICS CARE POINTS

- Prioritize sleep: Discuss with children and families the importance of sleep and make recommendations for healthy sleep including those listed above.
- Encourage families to limit duration of electronic media access as endorsed by AAP.
- Encourage families to limit or restrict electronic media access within 1 to 2 h of bedtime.
- Screen for sleep problems in youth with mood or behavioral problems, as insufficient sleep may be a contributing factor.
- For youth with sleep problems, ensure the steps above are observed before prescribing sleep medication.

DISCLOSURE

L. Hale has received consulting fees from Idorsia Pharmaceuticals and honoraria/travel support for lectures and consulting by various non-profits and universities. She ended her term as Editor-in-Chief of Sleep Health in 2020. T.A. Ceranoglu has received research support from Gerstner Family Foundation, United States Niraxx, Inc., Bee Foundation, United States The O'Sullivan Foundation, and is a member of board directors of Massachusetts Council on Gaming and Health.

REFERENCES

1. Council on Communications and Media. Media use in school-aged children and adolescents. Pediatrics 2016;138(5). https://doi.org/10.1542/peds.2016-2592.
2. Media CS. The Common Sense Census: Media Use by Tweens and Teens. 2019. Available at: https://www.commonsensemediaorg/research/the-common-sense-census-media-use-by-tweens-and-teens-2019.
3. Grandner MA, Fernandez FX. The translational neuroscience of sleep: a contextual framework. Science 2021;374(6567):568–73.
4. Astill RG, Van der Heijden KB, Van Ijzendoorn MH, et al. Sleep, cognition, and behavioral problems in school-age children: a century of research meta-analyzed. Psychol Bull 2012;138(6):1109–38.
5. Short MA, Blunden S, Rigney G, et al. Cognition and objectively measured sleep duration in children: a systematic review and meta-analysis. Sleep Health 2018; 4(3):292–300.

6. Reynaud E, Vecchierini MF, Heude B, et al. Sleep and its relation to cognition and behaviour in preschool-aged children of the general population: a systematic review. J Sleep Res 2018;27(3):e12636. https://doi.org/10.1111/jsr.12636.

7. Chaput JP, Gray CE, Poitras VJ, et al. Systematic review of the relationships between sleep duration and health indicators in the early years (0-4 years). BMC Publ Health 2017;17(Suppl 5):855.

8. Chaput JP, Gray CE, Poitras VJ, et al. Systematic review of the relationships between sleep duration and health indicators in school-aged children and youth. Appl Physiol Nutr Metab 2016;41(6 Suppl 3):S266–82.

9. Lampl M, Johnson ML. Infant growth in length follows prolonged sleep and increased naps. Sleep 2011;34(5):641–50.

10. Quist JS, Sjodin A, Chaput JP, et al. Sleep and cardiometabolic risk in children and adolescents. Sleep Med Rev 2016;29:76–100.

11. Meltzer LJ, Williamson AA, Mindell JA. Pediatric sleep health: it matters, and so does how we define it. Sleep Med Rev 2021;57:101425. https://doi.org/10.1016/j.smrv.2021.101425.

12. Hirshkowitz M, Whiton K, Albert SM, et al. National Sleep Foundation's updated sleep duration recommendations: final report. Sleep Health 2015;1(4):233–43.

13. Paruthi S, Brooks LJ, D'Ambrosio C, et al. Pediatric sleep duration consensus statement: a step forward. J Clin Sleep Med 2016;12(12):1705–6.

14. CDC. High School Students Sleep Data. Available at: https://www.cdc.gov/sleep/data-and-statistics/high-school-students.html.

15. Baiden P, Tadeo SK, Peters KE. The association between excessive screen-time behaviors and insufficient sleep among adolescents: Findings from the 2017 youth risk behavior surveillance system. Psychiatry Res 2019;281:112586. https://doi.org/10.1016/j.psychres.2019.112586.

16. Iglowstein I, Jenni OG, Molinari L, et al. Sleep duration from infancy to adolescence: reference values and generational trends. Pediatrics 2003;111(2):302–7.

17. Marciano L, Camerini AL. Recommendations on screen time, sleep and physical activity: associations with academic achievement in Swiss adolescents. Publ Health 2021;198:211–7.

18. Dworak M, Schierl T, Bruns T, et al. Impact of singular excessive computer game and television exposure on sleep patterns and memory performance of school-aged children. Pediatrics 2007;120(5):978–85.

19. Ivarsson M, Anderson M, Akerstedt T, et al. Playing a violent television game affects heart rate variability. Acta Paediatr 2009;98(1):166–72.

20. Ivarsson M, Anderson M, Akerstedt T, et al. The effect of violent and nonviolent video games on heart rate variability, sleep, and emotions in adolescents with different violent gaming habits. Psychosom Med 2013;75(4):390–6.

21. Weaver E, Gradisar M, Dohnt H, et al. The effect of presleep video-game playing on adolescent sleep. J Clin Sleep Med 2010;6(2):184–9.

22. King DL, Gradisar M, Drummond A, et al. The impact of prolonged violent video-gaming on adolescent sleep: an experimental study. J Sleep Res 2013;22(2):137–43.

23. T. C. Video games and sleep: an overlooked challenge. Adolesc Psychiatr 2014;4:104–8.

24. Brautsch LA, Lund L, Andersen MM, et al. Digital media use and sleep in late adolescence and young adulthood: a systematic review. Sleep Med Rev 2022;68:101742. https://doi.org/10.1016/j.smrv.2022.101742.

25. Cain N, Gradisar M. Electronic media use and sleep in school-aged children and adolescents: a review. Sleep Med 2010;11(8):735–42.

26. Duch H, Fisher EM, Ensari I, et al. Screen time use in children under 3 years old: a systematic review of correlates. Int J Behav Nutr Phys Act 2013;10:102.

27. Alonzo R, Hussain J, Stranges S, et al. Interplay between social media use, sleep quality, and mental health in youth: a systematic review. Sleep Med Rev 2021;56: 101414. https://doi.org/10.1016/j.smrv.2020.101414.

28. Hale L, Guan S. Screen time and sleep among school-aged children and adolescents: a systematic literature review. Sleep Med Rev 2015;21:50–8.

29. Carter B, Rees P, Hale L, et al. Association between portable screen-based media device access or use and sleep outcomes: a systematic review and meta-analysis. JAMA Pediatr 2016;170(12):1202–8.

30. Lund L, Solvhoj IN, Danielsen D, et al. Electronic media use and sleep in children and adolescents in western countries: a systematic review. BMC Publ Health 2021;21(1):1598.

31. Li X, Buxton OM, Lee S, et al. Sleep mediates the association between adolescent screen time and depressive symptoms. Sleep Med 2019;57:51–60.

32. Calamaro CJ, Mason TB, Ratcliffe SJ. Adolescents living the 24/7 lifestyle: effects of caffeine and technology on sleep duration and daytime functioning. Pediatrics 2009;123(6):e1005–10.

33. Chindamo S, Buja A, DeBattisti E, et al. Sleep and new media usage in toddlers. Eur J Pediatr 2019;178(4):483–90.

34. Guerrero MD, Barnes JD, Chaput JP, et al. Screen time and problem behaviors in children: exploring the mediating role of sleep duration. Int J Behav Nutr Phys Act 2019;16(1):105.

35. Rod NH, Dissing AS, Clark A, et al. Overnight smartphone use: a new public health challenge? A novel study design based on high-resolution smartphone data. PLoS One 2018;13(10):e0204811. https://doi.org/10.1371/journal.pone. 0204811.

36. Arora T, Broglia E, Thomas GN, et al. Associations between specific technologies and adolescent sleep quantity, sleep quality, and parasomnias. Sleep Med 2014; 15(2):240–7.

37. Scott H, Biello SM, Woods HC. Social media use and adolescent sleep patterns: cross-sectional findings from the UK millennium cohort study. BMJ Open 2019; 9(9):e031161. https://doi.org/10.1136/bmjopen-2019-031161.

38. Scott H, Biello SM, Woods HC. Identifying drivers for bedtime social media use despite sleep costs: the adolescent perspective. Sleep Health 2019;5(6):539–45.

39. Chang AM, Aeschbach D, Duffy JF, et al. Evening use of light-emitting eReaders negatively affects sleep, circadian timing, and next-morning alertness. Proc Natl Acad Sci U S A 2015;112(4):1232–7.

40. Perrault AA, Bayer L, Peuvrier M, et al. Reducing the use of screen electronic devices in the evening is associated with improved sleep and daytime vigilance in adolescents. Sleep 2019;42(9). https://doi.org/10.1093/sleep/zsz125.

41. Bartel K, Scheeren R, Gradisar M. Altering adolescents' pre-bedtime phone use to achieve better sleep health. Health Commun 2019;34(4):456–62.

42. Mahalingham T, Howell J, Clarke PJF. Assessing the effects of acute reductions in mobile device social media use on anxiety and sleep. J Behav Ther Exp Psychiatry 2023;78:101791. https://doi.org/10.1016/j.jbtep.2022.101791.

43. Rogers APB MK, Barber LK. Addressing FOMO and telepressure among university students: could a technology intervention help with social media use and sleep disruption? Comput Hum Behav 2019;93:192–9.

44. Exelmans L, Van den Bulck J. Bedtime, shuteye time and electronic media: sleep displacement is a two-step process. J Sleep Res 2017;26(3):364–70.

45. Haszard JJST, Smith C, Peddie MC, et al. Shuteye time compared with bedtime: MISCLASSIFICATION of sleep in adolescent females. J Measurement Physical Behav 2021;4:137–42.
46. van der Schuur WA, Baumgartner SE, Sumter SR. Social media use, social media stress, and sleep: examining cross-sectional and longitudinal relationships in adolescents. Health Commun 2019;34(5):552–9.
47. Jose PE, Vierling A. Cybervictimisation of adolescents predicts higher rumination, which in turn, predicts worse sleep over time. J Adolesc 2018;68:127–35.
48. Vernon L, Modecki KL, Barber BL. Tracking effects of problematic social networking on adolescent psychopathology: the mediating role of sleep disruptions. J Clin Child Adolesc Psychol 2017;46(2):269–83.
49. Vernon L, Barber BL, Modecki KL. Adolescent problematic social networking and school experiences: the mediating effects of sleep disruptions and sleep quality. Cyberpsychol Behav Soc Netw 2015;18(7):386–92.
50. Higuchi S, Motohashi Y, Liu Y, et al. Effects of playing a computer game using a bright display on presleep physiological variables, sleep latency, slow wave sleep and REM sleep. J Sleep Res 2005;14(3):267–73.
51. Twenge JM, Hisler GC, Krizan Z. Associations between screen time and sleep duration are primarily driven by portable electronic devices: evidence from a population-based study of U.S. children ages 0-17. Sleep Med 2019;56:211–8.
52. Hartmann M, Pelzl MA, Kann PH, et al. The effects of prolonged single night session of videogaming on sleep and declarative memory. PLoS One 2019;14(11): e0224893. https://doi.org/10.1371/journal.pone.0224893.
53. Green A, Cohen-Zion M, Haim A, et al. Evening light exposure to computer screens disrupts human sleep, biological rhythms, and attention abilities. Chronobiol Int 2017;34(7):855–65.
54. Chinoy ED, Duffy JF, Czeisler CA. Unrestricted evening use of light-emitting tablet computers delays self-selected bedtime and disrupts circadian timing and alertness. Physiol Rep 2018;6(10):e13692. https://doi.org/10.14814/phy2.13692.
55. Gronli J, Byrkjedal IK, Bjorvatn B, et al. Reading from an iPad or from a book in bed: the impact on human sleep. A randomized controlled crossover trial. Sleep Med 2016;21:86–92.
56. Schöllhorn I, Stefani O, Lucas RJ, et al. Melanopic irradiance defines the impact of evening display light on sleep latency, melatonin and alertness. Commun Biol 2023;6(1):228.
57. Higuchi S, Nagafuchi Y, Lee SI, et al. Influence of light at night on melatonin suppression in children. J Clin Endocrinol Metab 2014;99(9):3298–303.
58. Hartstein LE, Behn CD, Akacem LD, et al. High sensitivity of melatonin suppression response to evening light in preschool-aged children. J Pineal Res 2022;e12780. https://doi.org/10.1111/jpi.12780.
59. Eto T, Ohashi M, Nagata K, et al. Crystalline lens transmittance spectra and pupil sizes as factors affecting light-induced melatonin suppression in children and adults. Ophthalmic Physiol Opt 2021;41(4):900–10.
60. Hartstein LE, Diniz BC, Wright Jr KP, et al. Evening light intensity and phase delay of the circadian clock in early childhood. J Biol Rhythm 2022;38(1):77–86.
61. Heath M, Sutherland C, Bartel K, et al. Does one hour of bright or short-wavelength filtered tablet screenlight have a meaningful effect on adolescents' pre-bedtime alertness, sleep, and daytime functioning? Chronobiol Int 2014; 31(4):496–505.
62. Nagare R, Plitnick B, Figueiro M. Does the ipad night shift mode reduce melatonin suppression? Lighting Res Technol 2019;51(3):373–83.

63. Duraccio KM, Zaugg KK, Blackburn RC, et al. Does iPhone night shift mitigate negative effects of smartphone use on sleep outcomes in emerging adults? Sleep Health 2021;7(4):478–84.
64. Bowler J, Bourke P. Facebook use and sleep quality: light interacts with socially induced alertness. Br J Psychol 2019;110(3):519–29.
65. Robb MB. The new normal: parents, teens, screens, and sleep in the United States. Common Sense Media; 2019.
66. Murdock KK, Horissian M, Crichlow-Ball C. Emerging adults' text message use and sleep characteristics: a multimethod, naturalistic study. Behav Sleep Med 2017;15(3):228–41.
67. Scott H, Woods HC. Fear of missing out and sleep: cognitive behavioural factors in adolescents' nighttime social media use. J Adolesc 2018;68:61–5.
68. Wolfson AR, Carskadon MA, Acebo C, et al. Evidence for the validity of a sleep habits survey for adolescents. Sleep 2003;26(2):213–6.
69. Short MA, Gradisar M, Gill J, et al. Identifying adolescent sleep problems. PLoS One 2013;8(9):e75301.
70. Short MA, Gradisar M, Lack LC, et al. The discrepancy between actigraphic and sleep diary measures of sleep in adolescents. Sleep Med 2012;13(4):378–84.
71. Holley S, Hill CM, Stevenson J. A comparison of actigraphy and parental report of sleep habits in typically developing children aged 6 to 11 years. Behav Sleep Med 2010;8(1):16–27.
72. Weinstein E. The social media see-saw: positive and negative influences on adolescents' affective well-being. New Media Soc 2018;20(10):3597–623.
73. Paterson JL, Reynolds AC, Duncan M, et al. Barriers and enablers to modifying sleep behavior in adolescents and young adults: a qualitative investigation. Behav Sleep Med 2019;17(1):1–11.
74. Martin KB, Bednarz JM, Aromataris EC. Interventions to control children's screen use and their effect on sleep: a systematic review and meta-analysis. J Sleep Research 2021;30(3):e13130.
75. LeBourgeois MK, Hale L, Chang AM, et al. Digital media and sleep in childhood and adolescence. Pediatrics 2017;140(Suppl 2):S92–6.

Depression and Social Media Use in Children and Adolescents

Ailyn D. Diaz, MD[a],*, Dale Aaron Peeples, MD[b],
Paul E. Weigle, MD[c,d]

KEYWORDS

- Social media • Depression • Children • Adolescents • Parenting • Cyberbullying

KEY POINTS

- Adolescent depression rates have risen since 2007, coinciding with an explosive rise in social media engagement.
- A key to addressing depression related to social media use in youth is identifying problematic use and related depression via specific assessment tools.
- The family and home environment play a crucial role in shaping a child's social media interactions and resulting effect on mental health.
- Pediatricians are encouraged to adopt an approach that takes into account both clinical and developmental aspects in addressing social media use and depression.

INTRODUCTION

Ever since the inception of social media, youth have leveraged its capacity for connection with peers. The conceptualization of social media has undergone a significant expansion from its initial manifestation as a tool to share common interests with friends to its present iteration, incorporating greater capacity for user-created content dissemination, interpersonal communication, and community building.[1,2] Presently, social media platforms support engagement in diverse communities with complex layers of interaction among users, some using embedded artificial intelligence. This evolution in the capacities of social media platforms reflects a broader, more

[a] Division of Child and Adolescent Psychiatry, Department of Psychiatry and Behavioral Health, Pennsylvania State University College of Medicine, 500 University Drive, Hershey, PA 17033, USA; [b] Department of Psychiatry, Medical College of Georgia at Augusta University, 997 St. Sebastian Way, Augusta, GA 30912, USA; [c] Natchaug Hospital, Hartford Healthcare, 189 Storrs Avenue, Mansfield, CT 06250, USA; [d] Department of Psychiatry, UConn School of Medicine, 200 Academic Way, Farmington, CT 06032 USA
* Corresponding author.
E-mail address: adiaz@pennstatehealth.psu.edu

Pediatr Clin N Am 72 (2025) 175–187
https://doi.org/10.1016/j.pcl.2024.07.033   **pediatric.theclinics.com**

interactive digital landscape where children and youth are active participants with technology.

As the power and complexity of social media platforms has grown, so has engagement among youth: a staggering 95% of individuals aged 13 to 17 are active on social media, with 35% of them engaging with these platforms "almost constantly".[3] Notwithstanding the age restrictions imposed by regulations such as Children's Online Privacy Protection Rule (COPPA),[4] which sets the minimum user age of 13, there is a notable presence of younger children on social media platforms—38% between the ages of 8 and 12 use social media.[5] The deep integration of social media into the daily lives of youth coincides with critical periods of cognitive, socio-emotional learning, and physical development, and emerging data indicate that depression often manifests during these times.[6]

Rates of early-onset depression have climbed since late 2006 and can have lasting effects extending through adulthood, including low self-esteem, substance use, and difficulty maintaining healthy interpersonal relationships.[6,7] In the United States, 20.1% youth aged 12 to 17 experienced a major depressive episode in the past year, with 14.7% of those youth experiencing impairment in their ability to perform in school, complete chores at home, get along with others, and socialize.[8] A systematic review and meta-analysis of studies from 2004 to 2019 involving children younger than 13 estimated a far lower prevalence of 1.1% for depressive disorders.[9] Factors such as neuronal maturation and hormonal shifts during puberty and increasing dependency on complex interpersonal relationships may contribute to an increased incidence of depression during adolescence.[9,10] Early-onset depression is associated with more severe outcomes than adult depression, including suicide.[11] Twenty five percent of depressed adolescents suffer from severe depression, which is far more likely to be impairing and persist into adulthood.[12]

Pediatricians should understand complexities of the relationship between social media use and depressive symptoms. The current body of research lacks comprehensive longitudinal and experimental studies which would fully explain the manner in which social media affects youth through critical stages of childhood and adolescence. This article provides pediatricians with guidelines for evaluating depression in the setting of social media use including problematic use, identifying important factors that contribute to depression in social media use, and providing appropriate treatment.

The interplay between depression and social media in youth is complex, multifaceted, and not fully understood. Depression rates in adolescents have increased since 2007 correlating with the popularity of social media.[7] Youth who frequently use social media have higher rates of depression, which may be mediated by total entertainment screen time.[13] Conversely, those who spend more time in non-screen related activities, such as doing homework, reading print media, and attending church activities, report fewer mental health problems.[13] Recent increases in depression and suicide rates may be further explained by a generational shift toward screen time and away from engagement in non-screen activities.[13,14] Children ages 9 to 10 who use screen media over 2 hours a day are more likely than peers to experience symptoms of depression, engage in self-harm, think of suicide, or attempt suicide.[15] A recent meta-analysis demonstrated a small but significant association between screen time and depression.[16] The small magnitude of association might be indicative of the methods used in statistical analyses that focus on associations as opposed to relative risk, which considers the increased likelihood of depression occurring due to screen time.[17] Other studies have also found a significant association between depression and social media in those younger than 20 years of age but posit that social media use may benefit youth who are depressed (eg, by providing social support).[18]

Generational research confirms a closely-matching concomitant rise of social media and depression in the lives of American youth.[19] Studies of college students found that indices of mental health dropped at individual schools following the introduction of Facebook onto campus.[20] A wealth of correlational data confirms a modest link between time spent on social media and poor mental health among adolescents.[21] Longitudinal studies indicate that greater time spent on social media leads to a greater likelihood of new-onset depression 6 months later.[22] Combined, this evidence points to a strong link between social media use and depression. Randomized double-blind controlled trials of social media use would provide the best possible evidence but are impossible for 2 reasons: subjects cannot be blinded with regard to whether they are using social media and youth would not submit to instructions to use or refrain from social media on a daily basis for the extended periods needed for such studies to be useful. However, it seems improbable to imagine social media has an equal depressogenic effect on all users.

Research confirms that certain characteristics of the user and specific social media habits and experiences moderate this effect. Youth who tend toward social comparison, those with low social status, or are more likely to experience FOMO (fear of missing out) may be particularly likely to suffer depression with more time spent on social media.[23–26] Similarly, engaging with social media in a passive manner (looking at the posts of others without commenting or contributing themselves), those who multitasking with social media (eg, checking posts intermittently during schoolwork), have a problematic habit (compulsively checking social media excessively to the detriment of other activities), and those who use late at nighttime may be most subject to this effect.[27,28] Finally, youth involved in cyberbullying, as a bully or especially as a victim, may be most prone to depression.[29] Conversely, for youth enjoying high offline social support, using social media more may have a protective effect against depression. The displacement of in-person socializing, disruption of healthy sleep patterns, and decreased physical exercise due to excessive social media use could predispose individuals to depression. As we strive for a more nuanced understanding, it becomes imperative to consider the multifaceted interplay between specific online experiences, individual user characteristics, and the broader lifestyle implications of social media engagement in youth.

GENERAL ASSESSMENT OF SOCIAL MEDIA USE

An important step in managing depression in the context of social media use in children and adolescents is the identification of maladaptive, or problematic social media use and the underlying depressive state. Problematic social media use can be defined as an excessive habit which impairs functioning and is accompanied by symptoms associated with addiction (eg, withdrawal, tolerance, and dependence). Problematic use is associated with low self-esteem, low life satisfaction, depression, and loneliness, and may partially mediate the relationship between social media and depression.[30] Available screening tools may help assess problematic internet and social media use in clinical practice. It is important to take a holistic approach to assessment and screening, including an understanding of online habits and experiences.

A number of screening tools may assist in both the identification of problems and subsequently for assessment of treatment response. Several instruments have demonstrated validity in assessing problematic social media use in adolescents and young adults.[31] The Bergen Social Media Addiction Scale (BSMAS), the Social Media

Addiction Scale (SMAS), and the Social Media Disorders Scale (SMDS) are adapted from the Diagnostic and Statistical Manual (DSM) of Mental Disorders proposed criteria for internet gaming disorder, which are in turn modified criteria for substance use disorders and gambling disorder.[32–35] Broadly, these scales assess preoccupation, withdrawal, tolerance, displacement of other activities, inability to reduce use, excessive use, deception, and family conflict as a consequence of social media use.[35] All are short-form self-reports (6 to 10 items, answered yes/no or Likert scales), which take approximately 5 minutes to complete in a clinic. All were developed and tested internationally, demonstrating convergent validity to one another in a diverse group of age 13-19-year old American adolescents.[31] Among the scales, the BSMAS was shown to demonstrate better reliability in older adolescents.[31]

Problematic social media use, typically conceptualized as a behavioral addiction, may be accompanied by poor insight into problems associated with social media use. Patients and their families may object to the term problematic social media use due to implications of addiction. Therefore, assessing parental endorsement of symptoms is warranted, which can be evaluated via the Problematic Media Use Measure Short Form (PMUM-SF).[36] This instrument is not specific to social media, but rather overall screen engagement.[36]

Pediatricians may benefit from incorporating an assessment and discussion of social media use into initial patient encounters and follow-ups. Social media use is a major part of the lives of most adolescents, as a significant portion of an average teenager's day is spent on social media: connecting with peers, learning, and being entertained. Inquiry about this significant part of a child's life, which often has high consequences for self-esteem and well-being, is warranted. Helpful comprehensive guides to media assessment can be used to frame questions for assessment.[37] Many pediatricians currently incorporate the HEEADSSS (Home, Education, Eating, Activities, Drugs, Sexuality, Suicidal Ideation, and Safety) assessment model into adolescent wellness checks.[38] Incorporating a fourth S for Social Media is a helpful mnemonic.[39] See article 8-"Cracking the Algorithm: How to ask the right questions about social media during the interview" by Sood, Chapman, and Hadamati in this issue for more details about assessment of social media habits and experiences.

In brief, clinicians can initiate an open-ended discussion with patients about social media use. Such a discussion is most relevant to assessment of social history when discussing hobbies, peer relationships, and sexual history. Consider inquiring what platforms patients are most active on, an estimation of their time spent on social media, what they like and do not like about social media, the content of their social media feed, and household rules and expectations of social media use.

ASSESSMENT OF DEPRESSION

Screening and assessment of depression is a topic familiar to most pediatricians. Useful practice guidelines for assessing and managing depression are available from professional organizations, such as the American Academy of Pediatrics (AAP) and the American Academy of Child and Adolescent Psychiatry (AACAP).[40–42] Both documents were developed from a combination of expert consensus and evidence-based literature reviews. Most applicable to the practicing pediatrician is AAP's Guidelines for Adolescent Depression in Primary CARE (GLAD-PC), which focuses ages 10 to 21.[40,41] AACAP's Practice Parameters for depression are particularly beneficial, when considering best practices for assessment and management of younger children.[42]

GLAD-PC guidelines recommend annual screening for all adolescents aged 12 and older at annual visits, as well as screening children who have significant risk factors (eg, family history of mood disorder, childhood trauma or abuse, prior depression).[40,41] Clinicians are encouraged to consider evidence-based screening tools that are easy to administer and include self-report.[40,41] A good choice is the Patient Health Questionnaire-9 modified for adolescents (PHQ-9A), which assesses recent DSM criteria using a Likert scale and rates the severity of symptoms.[43]

AACAP practice guidelines also suggest universal screening in primary care for adolescents but not younger children.[42] When risk factors or symptoms suggest childhood depression, an appropriate screening tool is the Mood and Feelings Questionnaire (MFQ) offers both short and long-form versions for parents or children to complete.[44]

Screening for social media use in children and adolescents is a new clinical need and complicated by important limitations. Social media is rapidly evolving, and new and younger users may gravitate toward newer social media platforms. Consequently, screens normed in the past on an older social media platform like Facebook may not fully translate to the latest version of Facebook, much less to newer platforms (eg, TikTok). Many studies assessing screening measures focused on adolescents and young adults, and may not apply to children. Most screening measures attempt to detect problematic or addictive social media use, and may fail to capture the full impact of social media on young people's lives (eg, a teen who does not have addictive social media patterns but is significantly affected by cyberbullying). Future research should focus on updated screening of social media use across the lifespan, with measures for both parents and children.

MEDIATING FACTORS

The links between problematic social media use and depression are multi-factorial, with variation based on the individual's maturity and cognitive development, the nature of their social media habits and behaviors, the home environment, and social status. These may provide risks or protective factors to the individual child. Psychiatric co-morbidities influence the likelihood of problematic social media use and related depression. Some of the most important mediating factors follow.

Family and Friends

The family and home environment significantly shape if and how children engage with social media. Parents of children struggling with depression or other stressors often feel unable to limit their child's social media use or protect them from harm done by social media.[45] These parents are most likely to express inability to supervise whom their child communicates with, what they talk about, and when they do it.[45]

When treating adolescent depression, providers should empower parents to help children manage social media use. Parenting strategies broadly fall into categories of restriction (placing limits on use), active mediation (supporting the child's critical thinking about their use), and co-use (enjoying screen experiences together). Parents use different styles and approaches, and vary in permissiveness, expectations, warmth, and consistency with rules. A recent meta-analysis shows that positive parenting styles, such as authoritative style characterized by high warmth and involvement, may best prevent and address problematic internet use.[46] Beyens and colleagues found that restrictive approaches balanced to support adolescent autonomy may help reduce anxiety and depression, particularly when exacerbated by cyberbullying.[47] Parents who are open to adolescent input and discuss issues around media tend to have more success in helping children achieve healthy boundaries.[48]

Peers influence tends to grow as children move into adolescence. Adolescents enjoy greater autonomy in their social media use and engagement with peers. Social support can be protective against depression. For youth with high social status at school (who typically also have high social and support online) social media use may be protective against depression.[49] Social support gained via social media may be protective, but cannot replace offline relationships. One study found that youth high in offline social support were less likely to experience depressive symptoms than those with high online support or neither.[50] An adolescent's approach to social media can also affect risk for depression. Passive social media use, in which an adolescent monitors others' social media feeds without contributing (eg, no posting, 'liking' or commenting), has been associated with greater risk for depression, although inconsistently.[51] The nature of peer interactions on social media can greatly impact mood. Cyberbullying (ie, intentional, repeated, online harassment) is strongly associated with depression, as confirmed in a recent meta-analysis, especially for girls and older adolescents at highest risk.[52]

Sleep

Co-morbid issues explored thoroughly in this journal's companion articles (see article 1-"Social Media and Sleep Health" by Hale and colleagues, article 13-"Youth Digital Dilemmas: Exploring the Intersection Between Social Media and Anxiety" by Ariefdjohan and colleagues, and article 4-"The Impact of Social Media Use On the Development of Eating Disorders" by Gerwin and colleagues). However, it is worthwhile to briefly discuss the importance of insomnia, anxiety, and eating disorders in the relationship between depression and social media use. The impact of screen media on sleep is well documented, as inadequate sleep's capacity to predispose to and worsen depression. Screen media's impairment on sleep may be mediated by the physiologic impact of blue light from screens on melatonin release, interruption of sleep by notifications, arousal caused by engaging media content, and displacement of sleep time to engage with screen media. Many depressed youths retreat to their bedrooms after school, isolating and scrolling social media in bed in a "depressogenic" habit which runs contrary to their need for behavioral activation. Depression, social media use, and insomnia may evolve into a toxic feedback loop, in which depressed mood feeds into excessive social media engagement, worsening sleep, and consequently exacerbating depression.[53]

Anxiety

Anxiety and depression are common comorbidities. Depression can predispose toward anxiety and vice versa. Psychological stress related to social media experiences may in certain cases cause depression. Given the centrality of peer relationships to adolescents' self-esteem and well-being, adolescents who experience FOMO tend to increase engagement with social media, in doing so exacerbating their distress.[24] Similarly, adolescents may also fear they are being negatively judged and stress over management of their social media presence. The combination of FOMO and stress over curation of a social media presence may lead to compulsive social media use which is correlated with depression.[54]

Eating Disorders and Body Image

Social media has been shown to exacerbate negative body image via unfair comparisons with idealized images of peers, influencers, and celebrities.[42] Poor self-image negatively impacts well-being and can predispose to depression as well as eating disorders. Depression frequently accompanies eating disorders, a relationship mediated in part by the depressive effect of caloric restrictions.[43] Social media posts encouraging eating disordered behaviors trace back some of the earliest internet discussion boards and remain all too common today.

Treatment

Treatment guidelines for depression are outlined by the AAP and the AACAP.[40,42] In mild cases, monitoring, psychoeducation, and recommendations involving behavioral activation. In moderate to severe cases of depression, evidence-based interventions include psychotherapies based on Cognitive Behavioral Therapy (CBT) or Interpersonal Therapy (IPT).[42] Evidence-based pharmacologic strategies include the Selective Serotonin Reuptake Inhibitors, especially fluoxetine and escitalopram which are Food and Drug Administration-approved for treatment of depression in teens.[40,42] Familiarity with community resources for intensive therapeutic interventions and psychiatric care may be required for effective referrals of severe or refractory cases.

For youth at risk for problematic social media use, parental management of their online activity is warranted. Primary care providers must support children and families to sustain healthy and safe online habits. Means of doing so can be found online at the AAP's Center of Excellence on Social Media and Youth Mental Health and AACAP's Screen Media Resource Center. AAP's Family Media Plan, accessible through the Center of Excellence portal and at healthychildren.org, can be an excellent place to start in setting and maintaining health screen media habits which are personalized to the family's unique needs.[55] Setting up this plan enables families to clearly define about rules and expectations around media use, although a recent study found limited lasting changes after use.[55] Families may be most likely to benefit when a clinician initiates the media plan during an office visit, and subsequently follows up on its progress.[56]

Parents typically have greater influence over a child's access and interaction with social media than that of a teenager. Consequently, clinicians should encourage families to establish a media plan when children are young, and modify their parenting approach as a child matures, affording increasing agency to older children and teens in negotiating rules about media.[57] Parental control over time spent on social media in preadolescence is associated with reduced social media engagement, social comparisons, and depressive symptoms.[58] Parents should support appropriate adolescent autonomy by coming to agreement regarding limits on social media time and content.[47] Authoritarian, permissive, and uninvolved approaches should be avoided when possible.

Pediatricians can help prevent problematic use and depression by discussing healthy social media practices with patients and families. As a child begins to use social media, parents should have regular oversight and clearly define expectations around appropriate use while establishing firm limits on time and access. Parents should describe what behaviors on social media are unacceptable (eg, cruelty, sharing personal information, or sending sexually explicit pictures). Parents should explain to children that health information gained via social media is often unreliable, and discourage children from following social media posts focused on unhealthy behaviors such as drug use, self-harm, or eating disorders. Helping parents understand risks associated with social media use and encouraging them to consider limiting social media access may preclude subsequent impairment. Removing screen media from the bedroom entirely can prevent insomnia and enable better supervision. Teenagers typically respond better to a collaborative approach, balancing greater autonomy with appropriate limit setting, which should gradually fade as the teen demonstrates responsible use.[47,48,59]

ETHICAL CONCERNS

Pediatricians should be aware of the ethical considerations regarding social media use in youth with depression and their potential implications for parental supervision. Such considerations include balancing the child's needs for autonomy, peer engagement, self-expression, and privacy with the need to maintain healthy, safe social media habits. Research shows that depressed youth are more likely to overshare personal information via social media.[60] This may explain in part the higher risk depressed youth have of suffering cyberbullying, peer victimization, and exploitation via online contact with strangers.[52,61,62] Studies indicate that youth consider the most harmful uses of social media to be online risk taking, cyberbullying, negative social comparison, oversharing, posting negative updates, and encountering triggering material.[60]

The negative impacts of social media on psychological health raise ethical concerns about anonymity. Offered in varying degrees by social media platforms, anonymity may enable destructive interactions such as cyberbullying and online discrimination (ie, racially motivated bias enacted on social media).[63,64] Black youth are at a heightened risk of encountering online discrimination, which may involve hate imagery, derogatory comments, or harmful acts.[64,65] Research findings indicate personal experiences of discrimination are directly associated with depression, even when controlling for racial identity, gender, discrimination encountered offline, and perceived stress levels.[63]

Pediatricians may also find that young patients who acknowledge the risks associated with sharing self-harm behaviors on social media still partake in such actions for the sake of validation and connection. Children and adolescents frequently falsify their age to gain access to social media sites, which parents should discourage.[66] The American Academy of Pediatrics encourages the minimum user age of 13 set by COPPA.[4,66] Pediatricians should encourage parents to be aware of their children's social media use, limit and supervise internet access, offer guidance on social media safety, and convey the importance of a healthy balance between online interactions and real-world relationships.

SOCIAL MEDIA AND HELP-SEEKING IN DEPRESSION

Social media offers opportunity for support for those struggling with depression. It offers a unique means for connecting struggling individuals with supportive peers. Social media platforms have made limited efforts to de-platform or censor content that graphically depicts self-harm or suicide, and promote messages of hope and recovery support.[67] Critical crisis intervention resources area available for those flagged as in need by those concerned about their social media posts. Youth with depression often report finding helpful self-expression, community, and inspiration via social media.

Youth use social media as a tool to obtain health information and support. In a systematic study of young people aged 12 to 25, many reported finding value to gathering health-related information from social media hence considering these platforms beneficial.[68] Social media can facilitate social inclusion, especially for youth who identify as Lesbian, Gay, Bisexual, Transgender, Queer, Intersex and Asexual and are at risk for depression due to social isolation.[69] Finding acceptance and validation in like-minded communities on social media can help restore self-esteem and psychological well-being.[70]

SUMMARY

Pediatricians should understand how various aspects of social media engagement affect depression. Providers should evaluate the social media habits and experience of their patients, especially those who suffer depression. Pediatricians can provide guidance to parents and children on navigating the challenges posed by social media, moderating use, and minimizing its potential negative effects. Further longitudinal research is needed to assess how social media influences depression in adolescents. Pediatricians should stay abreast with evolving evidence-based practices to identify and address social media use, depression, and their interactions in young patients. Social media companies should work with pediatricians and child psychiatrists to produce features that maximize healthy use and experiences and eliminate harmful elements. Pediatricians should support efforts to hold social media companies liable for mental health damage done by their platforms, in order to incentivize such changes. A comprehensive and collaborative effort is essential to help children and adolescents circumvent depression and thrive during the mental health crisis of our digital age.

CLINICS CARE POINTS

- Recommend a family screen media plan which is regularly revisited and revised.
- Advise parents to strongly consider banning screen media from the dinner table and from the bedrooms of children and teens, especially at night.
- Encourage parents of children and less mature teens who use social media to consider regular checks of social media content.[55]
- Clinicians should increase their knowledge of social media functions and material popular with children to better evaluate patients' use and guide families.
- Clinicians should advise parents of depressed youth to encourage behavioral activation by scheduling healthy activities such as in-person socialization, outings, active hobbies, and exercise, while minimizing inactivity and screen time.

DISCLOSURE

The authors have no disclosures.

REFERENCES

1. Burgess J, Marwick A, Poell T. The SAGE handbook of social media. SAGE Publications Ltd; 2018. Available at: https://sk.sagepub.com/reference/the-sage-handbook-of-social-media.
2. Aichner T, Grünfelder M, Maurer O, et al. Twenty-five years of social media: A review of social media applications and definitions from 1994 to 2019. Cyberpsychol, Behav Soc Netw 2021;24(4):215–22.
3. Pew Research Center. Teens, social media, and technology. 2022. Available at: https://www.pewresearch.org/internet/2022/08/10/teens-social-media-and-technology-2022/.
4. FTC. Children's Online Privacy Protection Rule. In: Commission FT, editor. Washington D.C.1998.
5. Rideout V, Peebles A, Mann S, et al. Common Sense census: media use by tweens and teens. San Francisco, California: Common Sense; 2021.

6. Solmi M, Radua J, Olivola M, et al. Age at onset of mental disorders worldwide: large-scale meta-analysis of 192 epidemiological studies. Mol Psychiatr 2022; 27(1):281–95.

7. Geiger AW, Davis L. A growing number of American teenagers – particularly girls – are facing depression. Teens & Youth blog; 2019–. Available at: https://www. pewresearch.org/short-reads/2019/07/12/a-growing-number-of-american-teenagers-particularly-girls-are-facing-depression/#:~:text=The%20number%20of%20adults %20who,5%25%20of%20men.

8. Substance Abuse and Mental Health Services Administration. Key substance use and mental health indicators in the United States: Results from the 2021 National Survey on Drug Use and Health. 2022. 37–38. Available at: https://www.samhsa. gov/data/report/2021-nsduh-annual-national-report.

9. Spoelma MJ, Sicouri GL, Francis DA, et al. Estimated Prevalence of Depressive Disorders in Children From 2004 to 2019: A Systematic Review and Meta-Analysis. JAMA Pediatr 2023;177(10):1017–27.

10. Bakker MP, Ormel J, Verhulst FC, et al. Peer stressors and gender differences in adolescents' mental health: the TRAILS study. J Adolesc Health 2010;46(5): 444–50.

11. Mangione CM, Barry MJ, Nicholson WK, et al. Screening for depression and suicide risk in children and adolescents: US preventive services task force recommendation statement. JAMA 2022;328(15):1534–42.

12. Avenevoli S, Swendsen J, He J-P, et al. Major Depression in the National Comorbidity Survey–Adolescent Supplement: Prevalence, Correlates, and Treatment. J Am Acad Child Adolesc Psychiatr 2015-01-01 2015;54(1):37–44.e2.

13. Twenge JM, Joiner TE, Rogers ML, et al. Increases in depressive symptoms, suicide-related outcomes, and suicide rates among U.S. adolescents after 2010 and links to increased new media screen time. Clin Psychol Sci 2018; 6(1):3–17.

14. Haidt J, Allen N. Scrutinizing the effects of digital technology on mental health. Nature 2020;7794:226–7.

15. Roberston L, Twenge JM, Joiner TE, et al. Associations between screen time and internalizing disorder diagnoses among 9- to 10-year-olds. J Affect Disord 2022; 311:530–7.

16. Ivie EJ, Pettitt A, Moses LJ, et al. A meta-analysis of the association between adolescent social media use and depressive symptoms. J Affect Disord 2020; 275:165–74.

17. Twenge JM, Hamilton JL. Linear correlation is insufficient as the sole measure of associations: The case of technology use and mental health. Acta Psychol 2022; 229:103696.

18. Arias-de la Torre J, Puigdomenech E, García X, et al. Relationship between depression and the use of mobile technologies and social media among adolescents: Umbrella review. J Med Internet Res 2020;22(8):e16388.

19. Twenge JM. Generations: the real differences between Gen Z, Millennials, Gen X, Boomers, and Silents–and what they mean for America's future. In: First atria books hardcover edition. Atria Books; 2023.

20. Braghieri L, Levy RE, Makarin A. Social Media and Mental Health. Am Econ Rev 2022;112(11):3660–93.

21. Valkenburg PM, Meier A, Beyens I. Social media use and its impact on adolescent mental health: An umbrella review of the evidence. Curr Opin Psychol 2022;44:58–68.

22. Primack BA, Bisbey MA, Shensa A, et al. The association between valence of social media experiences and depressive symptoms. Depress Anxiety 2018;35(8): 784–94.
23. Handbook of adolescent digital media use and mental health. Cambridge University Press; 2022.
24. Beyens I, Frison E, Eggermont S. "I don't want to miss a thing": Adolescents' fear of missing out and its relationship to adolescents' social needs, Facebook use, and Facebook related stress. Comput Hum Behav 2016;64:1–8.
25. Zheng Z, Liu W, Yang L, et al. Group Differences: The Relationship between Social Media Use and Depression during the Outbreak of COVID-19 in China. Int J Environ Res Publ Health 2022;19(21):13941.
26. Lopes LS, Valentini JP, Monteiro TH, et al. Problematic Social Media Use and Its Relationship with Depression or Anxiety: A Systematic Review. Cyberpsychol, Behav Soc Netw 2022;25(11):691–702.
27. Valkenburg PM, Van Driel II, Beyens I. The associations of active and passive social media use with well-being: A critical scoping review. New Media Soc 2022-02-01 2022;24(2):530–49.
28. Chen Q, Yan Z. Does multitasking with mobile phones affect learning? A review. Comput Hum Behav 2016;54:34–42.
29. Völlink T, Bolman CAW, Dehue F, et al. Coping with Cyberbullying: Differences Between Victims, Bully-victims and Children not Involved in Bullying. J Community Appl Soc Psychol 2013;23(1):7–24.
30. Huang C. A meta-analysis of the problematic social media use and mental health. Int J Soc Psychiatr 2022;68(1):12–33.
31. Watson JC, Prosek EA, Giordano AL. Investigating Psychometric Properties of Social Media Addiction Measures Among Adolescents. J Counsel Dev 2020; 98(4):458–66.
32. Andreassen CS, Torsheim T, Brunborg GS, et al. Development of a Facebook Addiction Scale. Psychol Rep 2012;110(2):501–17.
33. van den Eijnden RJJM, Lemmens JS, Valkenburg PM. The Social Media Disorder Scale. Comput Hum Behav 2016;61:478–87.
34. Şahin C. Social Media Addiction Scale-Student Form: The Reliability and Validity Study. Turkish Online Journal of Educational Technology 2018;17:169–82.
35. American Psychiatric Association. Conditions for Further Study. Diagnostic and Statistical Manual of Mental Disorders 2022.
36. Domoff SE, Harrison K, Gearhardt AN, et al. Development and validation of the Problematic Media Use Measure: A parent report measure of screen media "addiction" in children. Psychology of Popular Media Culture 2019;8(1):2–11.
37. Carson NJ, Gansner M, Khang J. Assessment of Digital Media Use in the Adolescent Psychiatric Evaluation. Child and Adolescent Psychiatric Clinics of North America 2018;27(2):133–43.
38. Doukrou M, Segal TY. Fifteen-minute consultation: Communicating with young people-how to use HEEADSSS, a psychosocial interview for adolescents. Arch Dis Child Educ Pract Ed 2018;103(1):15–9.
39. Clark DL, Raphael JL, McGuire AL. HEADS4: Social Media Screening in Adolescent Primary Care. Pediatrics 2018;141(6). https://doi.org/10.1542/peds.2017-3655.
40. Cheung AH, Zuckerbrot RA, Jensen PS, et al. GLAD-PC STEERING GROUP. Guidelines for Adolescent Depression in Primary Care (GLAD-PC): Part II. Treatment and Ongoing Management. Pediatrics 2018;141(3). https://doi.org/10.1542/peds.2017-4082.

41. Zuckerbrot RA, Cheung A, Jensen PS, et al. GLAD-PC STEERING GROUP. Guidelines for Adolescent Depression in Primary Care (GLAD-PC): Part I. Practice Preparation, Identification, Assessment, and Initial Management. Pediatrics 2018;141(3). https://doi.org/10.1542/peds.2017-4081.

42. Walter HJ, Abright AR, Bukstein OG, et al. Clinical Practice Guideline for the Assessment and Treatment of Children and Adolescents With Major and Persistent Depressive Disorders. J Am Acad Child Adolesc Psychiatry 2023;62(5): 479–502.

43. Richardson LP, McCauley E, Grossman DC, et al. Evaluation of the Patient Health Questionnaire-9 Item for detecting major depression among adolescents. Pediatrics 2010;126(6):1117–23.

44. Angold A, Costello E, Messer S, et al. The Development of a Questionnaire for Use in Epidemiological Studies of Depression in Children and Adolescents. Int J Methods Psychiatr Res 1995;5:237–49.

45. Lewis AJ, Knight T, Germanov G, et al. The Impact on Family Functioning of Social Media Use by Depressed Adolescents: A Qualitative Analysis of the Family Options Study. Front Psychiatr 2015;6:131.

46. Niu X, Li JY, King DL, et al. The relationship between parenting styles and adolescent problematic Internet use: A three-level meta-analysis. J Behav Addict 2023; 12(3):652–69.

47. Beyens I, Keijsers L, Coyne SM. Social media, parenting, and well-being. Curr Opin Psychol 2022;47:101350.

48. Dingus Keuhlen K, Donald K, Falbo R, et al. Stop! Collaborate and Listen: A Content Analysis of Peer-Reviewed Articles Investigating Parenting Strategies for Managing Adolescent Internet Use. Contemp Fam Ther 2020;42. https://doi. org/10.1007/s10591-019-09510-z.

49. Huang C. Correlations of online social network size with well-being and distress: A meta-analysis. Cyberpsychology 2021;15(2). https://doi.org/10.5817/cp2021-2-3.

50. Longest K, Kang J-A. Social Media, Social Support, and Mental Health of Young Adults During COVID-19. Frontiers in Communication 2022;7. https://doi.org/10. 3389/fcomm.2022.828135.

51. Frison E, Eggermont S. Exploring the Relationships Between Different Types of Facebook Use, Perceived Online Social Support, and Adolescents' Depressed Mood. Soc Sci Comput Rev 2016;34(2):153–71.

52. Hu Y, Bai Y, Pan Y, et al. Cyberbullying victimization and depression among adolescents: A meta-analysis. Psychiatr Res 2021;305:114198.

53. Przepiorka A, Blachnio A. The Role of Facebook Intrusion, Depression, and Future Time Perspective in Sleep Problems Among Adolescents. J Res Adolesc 2020;30(2):559–69.

54. Dhir A, Yossatorn Y, Kaur P, et al. Online social media fatigue and psychological wellbeing—A study of compulsive use, fear of missing out, fatigue, anxiety and depression. Int J Inf Manag 2018;40:141–52.

55. American Academy of Pediatrics. How to make a family media use plan. healthychildren.org. Available at: https://www.healthychildren.org/English/family-life/ Media/Pages/How-to-Make-a-Family-Media-Use-Plan.aspx?gad_source=1&gclid= CjwKCAiA75itBhA6EiwAkho9e58_QZtaLmZrTJeE9J6BKwWU1L3vRSUB24W_t9p 9zXLFd_1ZdoFHnRoCyWkQAvD_BwE. [Accessed 16 January 2024].

56. Moreno MA, Binger KS, Zhao Q, et al. Effect of a Family Media Use Plan on Media Rule Engagement Among Adolescents: A Randomized Clinical Trial. JAMA Pediatr 2021;175(4):351–8.

57. Young R, Tully M. Autonomy vs. control: Associations among parental mediation, perceived parenting styles, and U. S. adolescents' risky online experiences. Cyberpsychology 2022;16(2):Article 5.
58. Fardouly J, Magson NR, Johnco CJ, et al. Parental Control of the Time Preadolescents Spend on Social Media: Links with Preadolescents' Social Media Appearance Comparisons and Mental Health. J Youth Adolesc 2018;47(7):1456–68.
59. Dawson RS. Talking to Adolescents About Social Media. Pediatr Ann 2017;46(8):e274–6.
60. Radovic A, Gmelin T, Stein BD, et al. Depressed adolescents' positive and negative use of social media. J Adolesc 2017;55:5–15.
61. Frison E, Subrahmanyam K, Eggermont S. The Short-Term Longitudinal and Reciprocal Relations Between Peer Victimization on Facebook and Adolescents' Well-Being. J Youth Adolesc 2016;45(9):1755–71.
62. Forni G, Pietronigro A, Tiwana N, et al. Little red riding hood in the social forest. Online grooming as a public health issue: a narrative review. Ann Ig 2020;32(3):305–18.
63. Tynes BM, Giang MT, Williams DR, et al. Online racial discrimination and psychological adjustment among adolescents. J Adolesc Health 2008;43(6):565–9.
64. Tynes BM, Rose CA, Williams DR. The development and validation of the online victimization scale for adolescents. Cyberpsychology 2010;4(2).
65. Del Toro J, Wang MT. online racism and mental health among black American adolescents in 2020. J Am Acad Child Adolesc Psychiatry 2023;62(1):25–36.e8.
66. O'Keeffe GS, Clarke-Pearson K, Council on Communications and Media. The impact of social media on children, adolescents, and families. Pediatrics 2011;127(4):800–4.
67. Google. Suicide, self-harm, and eating disorders policy. YouTube. Available at: https://support.google.com/youtube/answer/2802245?hl=en. [Accessed 16 January 2024].
68. Pretorius C, Chambers D, Coyle D. Young People's Online Help-Seeking and Mental Health Difficulties: Systematic Narrative Review. J Med Internet Res 2019;21(11):e13873.
69. McDonald K. Social Support and Mental Health in LGBTQ Adolescents: A review of the literature. Issues Ment Health Nurs 2018;39(1):16–29.
70. Berger MN, Taba M, Marino JL, et al. Social Media Use and Health and Well-being of Lesbian, Gay, Bisexual, Transgender, and Queer Youth: Systematic Review. Review. J Med Internet Res 2022;24(9):e38449.

Understanding Adolescent Self-esteem and Self-image Through Social Media Behaviors

Linda Charmaraman, PhD[a],*, Horacio Hojman, MD, MBA[b],
Jenni Quichimbo Auqui, BA[a], Zhamilya Bilyalova[a]

KEYWORDS

- Adolescent self-esteem • Online social comparisons • Online self-presentation
- Body image • Selfies • Normative narcissism • Appearance-contingent self-worth

KEY POINTS

- In understanding self-esteem and self-image in adolescence, it is imperative to keep in mind normative adolescent identity development and how adolescents present themselves to society in the online world as well as their online interactions on social media.
- Adolescents may use social media accounts to emotionally regulate self-esteem and self-image which may be related to their levels of anxiety, depression, and loneliness, with studies showing that social media can either positively or negatively affect self-esteem.
- As a normative part of adolescent social comparison seeking, adolescents may build their self-esteem and self-image through social feedback, accepting or rejecting interactions with online peers. As society is more focused on female physical appearance, appearance-contingent self-worth is found more frequently in females.
- Selfies, a social media form of self-portraiture have become a powerful means for self-expression in adolescents, identifying with idealized figures toward their own separation-individuation from primary parental figures.
- Rather than making sweeping generalizations about negative outcomes related to youth social media use, in clinical practice it is important to consider intersectional identity factors of a particular youth when assessing impacts of social media on self-esteem.

INTRODUCTION

A key factor in youth well-being during adolescence is self-esteem, which is shaped by an individual's social environment. Positive social interactions with others are associated with higher self-esteem.[1] One of the most prominent changes during

[a] Youth, Media, & Wellbeing Research Lab, Wellesley Centers for Women, Wellesley College, 106 Central Street, Wellesley, MA 02481, USA; [b] Department of Psychiatry and Human Behavior, Alpert Medical School, Brown University, Providence, RI 02912, USA
* Corresponding author. Wellesley Centers for Women, 106 Central Street, Wellesley, MA 02481.
E-mail address: lcharmar@wellesley.edu

Pediatr Clin N Am 72 (2025) 189–201
https://doi.org/10.1016/j.pcl.2024.07.034
pediatric.theclinics.com
0031-3955/25/© 2024 Elsevier Inc. All rights are reserved, including those for text and data mining, AI training, and similar technologies.

this developmental period is the adoption of new social technologies throughout early (age 10–14) and late (15–19) adolescence. In this article, self-esteem and self-image during the adolescent years in the digital age will be discussed concerning several interrelated factors, including social media influences, normative developmental stages, peer influence, loneliness, online self-presentation, social comparisons, narcissism, contingent self-worth, and body image.

THE RISE OF SOCIAL MEDIA IN ADOLESCENCE

The prevalence and impact of social media on today's youth, especially adolescents, cannot be overstated. Recent data from a survey conducted by Pew Research Center in 2023 show that platforms like YouTube, TikTok, Instagram, and Snapchat are widely used by teens.[2] In recent years, there has been a notable increase in screen time among teens and tweens according to Common Sense Media in 2021.[3] For example, during school hours, the app categories that took up the highest proportion of time were social media (32% of smartphone use during school hours), gaming (17%), and YouTube (26%). What is particularly concerning is the rise in social media use among children aged 8 to 12, despite age restrictions. YouTube is the platform most commonly used by teens, with 95% of those ages 13 to 17 saying they have ever used it. Two-thirds of teens report using TikTok, followed by roughly 6-in-10 who say they use Instagram (62%) and Snapchat (59%). Much smaller shares of teens say they have ever used Twitter (23%), Twitch (20%), WhatsApp (17%), Reddit (14%) and Tumblr (5%). Gender differences are also evident, with teen girls engaging more on platforms like TikTok, Instagram, and Snapchat, while boys lean toward YouTube, Twitch, and Reddit.[4] TikTok use is particularly more common among black teens and among teen girls. The survey reveals that many teens find it challenging to give up social media and report both positive (feeling connected, expressing creativity) and negative (feeling overwhelmed, peer pressure) experiences. Importantly, these findings emphasize the need to delve deeper into how social media affects the self-esteem of youth, especially teens who are already at risk or dealing with mental health challenges because they are both more likely to have negative experiences with social media and value the benefits of social media, like finding resources, community, or support.[5]

SELF-ESTEEM, SELF-PRESENTATION, AND NORMATIVE ADOLESCENT IDENTITY DEVELOPMENT

Perhaps the most widely accepted definition of self-esteem stems from Rosenberg[6] who defines self-esteem as one's subjective view of oneself. Recent psychologists have further elaborated the definition of self-esteem by underlining the differences between self-esteem and similar concepts such as self-evaluation.[1] Adolescent self-esteem presents itself across various domains of self-worth including athletic, academic, social, and physical characteristics of oneself. A systematic review revealed that social media promotes adolescent identity development by satisfying their need for relatedness, competence, and autonomy.[7] Vogel and colleagues[8] conceptualize self-esteem as both a mostly stable trait that develops over time and a fluid state that is responsive to daily events and contexts. Social media influences adolescent identity development in different ways. Adolescents tend to experience social pressure, the Fear of Missing out or FOMO, or negative peer feedback which may harm the formation of their identity and negatively impact self-esteem.[7] In a study by Quatman and Watson,[9] assessing 10 measures of self-esteem among 545 adolescents in the 8th, 10th, and 12th grade, the researchers found that boys scored higher on global self-esteem and almost all other domains of self-esteem than girls.[10] In fact, research finds that during adolescence, self-esteem drops twice as much for girls compared to boys.[11] Some explanations offered for the significant drop in self-esteem for girls include biological and cognitive changes as well as larger societal expectations for women.[11] In a study by Adams and colleagues,[12] the researchers found that African American participants were more likely to report high self-esteem than European American participants and Hispanic participants. The researchers hypothesized that African American participants may have exhibited higher levels of self-esteem because of a strong ethnic pride and sense of community.[12]

Online self-presentation is the process in creating an outward-facing self-concept in adolescents, a key developmental task during the adolescent period.[13] Self-concept refers to one's overall perception of oneself, including one's memories. Self-presentation behaviors promote self-concept formation by inviting public feedback on one's exploratory self-presentations that then may result in the desire to maintain, adjust, or escape from that presentation.[14] Besides being an entertainment tool (scrolling/watching content on Instagram, Tiktok, etc), social networks allow users to construct electronic profiles for themselves in which they can provide details about their lives and experiences, post pictures, maintain relationships, plan social events, meet new people, make observations of others' lives, fulfill belongingness needs, and express their beliefs, preferences, and emotions.[8] Adolescents who focus on attaining positive and realistic possible selves are generally more likely to report higher levels of self-esteem than those who focus on negative or unrealistic selves.[15] When adolescents present themselves via social media before developing a stable self-concept, they often present multiple highly idealized selves than those who reported a more fully defined self-concept. For instance, Balick[16] describes the "false self" as the vehicle for our self-expression on status updates and tweets. In this way, the individual protects aspects of subjectivities that are less positive and happy to be projected into the world. Online self-presentation can also facilitate positive effects on the development of self-concept as adolescents interact with others through comments and messages, potentially resulting in the formation of supportive online peer groups. Studies have documented effective interventions to enhance self-esteem, such as in a study of resilience and cultural identity, researchers found that a culturally grounded program for indigenous youth increased levels of cultural self-esteem.[17]

IMPORTANCE OF SELF-ESTEEM AND CONNECTING WITH PEERS IN DIGITAL ENVIRONMENTS

Researchers have suggested that self-esteem may be affected by both incidental and long-term exposure to social media.[8] Positive and negative experiences on social media predict the amount of time spent on social media, but more importantly, can predict changes in self-esteem.[18] Conversely, self-esteem may impact the way adolescents engage with social media. When young adolescent girls were asked what general social media guidance they tend to seek from adults or peers, the most frequently mentioned topic is to improve their self-esteem, as opposed to getting less hooked on social media or avoiding harms.[19] Studies find that individuals with low self-esteem are more likely to shy away from actively engaging in social media platforms like posting content.[20] Nonetheless, individuals with low self-esteem tend to engage in the act of "lurking" which involves keeping track of people.[20] Those with a high self-esteem on average but fluctuate up and down due to external circumstances report fewer positive social media experiences compared to their peers and may be particularly vulnerable to a drop in self-esteem due to negative online experiences.[18] While some studies argue that social media may negatively affect self-esteem, in a study by Mackson and colleagues[21] the researchers found that self-esteem can be positively associated with social media use. They found that participants with Instagram accounts reported higher levels of self-esteem and lower levels of anxiety, depression, and loneliness compared to non-users. Effects of social media may also depend on individual characteristics that they bring such that adolescents with low self-esteem have been found to have positive effects in self-esteem the longer they spend on social media compared to adolescents with average self-esteem.[18]

Researchers have found that social self-esteem is related to how adolescents engage with peers on social media sites,[22] particularly when adolescence is a developmental period that centers around peer influence. Peer relationships in real life often mirror their social relationships in the online world. For instance, high self-esteem is linked to more online friends. Many adolescents engage in social media to seek acceptance and popularity.[23] Not only do adolescents build a social rapport via social media use, but they also develop their identities.[7] This sense of identity is often fueled by a sense of belonging in groups with which an adolescent relates to.[24] Using social media has been shown to strengthen a sense of belonging in a community for older teenagers, particularly those with low self-esteem.[25]

Social media use has been related not only to greater social connectedness and well-being, but also to increased loneliness. Loneliness is defined as a unique condition in which an individual perceives himself or herself to be socially isolated even when among other people. Loneliness is a subjective psychological state, and has been associated with objective social isolation, depression, introversion, or poor social skills.[26] For instance, Pop and colleagues[27] found that the use of Snapchat was found to be strongly positively correlated with self-esteem in a study of medical students. Almost half of the students demonstrated an association between Snapchat use and a moderate to high level of loneliness. Age and gender were found to be important; the younger the user, the higher the scores for loneliness and feeling depressed, and the greater the number of hours on social networks. In contrast, prior research has also demonstrated that adolescents use social media to reduce feelings of isolation and loneliness. For instance, black, Latine, and LGBTQ and youth are significantly more likely to use online communities to reduce social isolation compared to their white and heteronormative peers.[28]

Due to the mixed findings of the relationship between self-esteem and social media use, a systematic review found that social media does not significantly impact the self-esteem of the majority of users but rather that there are person-specific factors based on individual susceptibilities, strengths, specific motivations, and types of use.[29] Rather than making sweeping generalizations about negative outcomes related to youth social media use, in clinical practice it is important to consider intersectional identity factors of a particular youth when assessing impacts of social media.

ONLINE SOCIAL COMPARISONS

Adolescence in particular is a time in which social comparisons become more important to individuals. Adolescents see peer interactions as an increasingly integral and rewarding part of their lives and they invest more in friendships during this time. They also move from primarily seeking adult affirmation in childhood to valuing the input of their peers above that of adults during adolescence.[24] Krause and colleagues[30] find that the 3 processes that drive self-esteem are: 1. social feedback processing, defined as a process that involves one's ability to self-evaluate depending on the accepting or rejecting nature of interactions with others, 2. social comparison, defined as the need for individuals to assess themselves by taking into consideration others' evaluations of their capabilities,[31] and 3. self-reflection, defined as an individual's reflection of items like one's previous behavior.[32] Social comparison is a normative aspect of adolescent development serving affiliation needs, facilitating decision-making, and helping regulate positive and negative emotions.[8] Social comparison promotes self-concept development as it helps individuals learn about themselves and increases their motivation to engage in self-enhancement and self-evaluation and criticism. Because adolescents formulate their self-concepts based on the opinions and actions of others, online social comparisons may further influence their development of self. Females generally report feared possible selves (eg, fears regarding one's future self) pertaining to interpersonal relationships and anticipate the reality of feared selves more so than males.[13] Upward social comparison occurs when comparing oneself with others they perceive as superior or having more social capital,[33] whereas downward social comparison occurs when comparing oneself with others with less social status. Although upward comparison can be beneficial when it inspires people to become more like their comparison targets, having primarily upward comparisons online more often produces feelings of inadequacy, poorer self-evaluation, and experiencing negative affect.[8]

Adolescents, in particular, may be vulnerable to critical self-views facilitated by these upwards social comparisons, since adolescents increasingly rely on their peer contexts to inform their self-views. Adolescents move from a childhood overly optimistic or grandiose assessment of self to more accurate but less positive assessment of themselves during adolescence. Increased social comparisons and awareness of peer contexts may be one of the reasons for this shift in self-image. A recent study noted that Instagram users who reported higher levels of social anxiety, also had a higher Instagram-contingent self-worth, which was displayed via behaviors like consistently editing post captions.[34] Meier and colleagues suggest that comparing oneself upwards on social networking sites (SNSs) can also lead to positive outcomes, such as feeling inspired, which is closely linked to well-being. When users encounter highly positive and curated nature and travel posts on Instagram, they tend to engage in stronger upward comparisons, resulting in feelings of inspiration through a benign envy reaction, ultimately boosting their well-being.

SELFIES AND NARCISSISM

Social media sites can be convenient opportunities for those who seek appraisals and crave admiration from others. Narcissism has been strongly associated with high self-esteem as well as unstable self-esteem.[35] In a meta-analysis of 80 studies,[20] researchers have demonstrated that higher social media use was significantly associated with lower levels of self-esteem, higher loneliness, and higher narcissism, particularly in non-Western, non-individualistic countries. They also found that high levels of narcissism are highly associated with any type of active social media use, including total number of friends, commenting/liking posts, posting photos, and status updates. There is growing evidence to suggest that there are at least 2 forms of trait narcissism, namely grandiose narcissism and vulnerable narcissism. Grandiose narcissism, often referred to as "textbook" narcissism, is the most well-known form of narcissism and is characterized by high self-esteem, extraversion, confidence, and social boldness. Vulnerable narcissism, also referred to as hypersensitive, covert, fragile, or implicit narcissism is in stark contrast to the self-assuredness of grandiose narcissism. Vulnerable narcissism is characterized by hypersensitivity to the opinions of others, an intense desire for approval, defensiveness, low self-esteem, introversion, neuroticism, and insecurity, which is more commonly found when one uses social media in a passive way (eg, lurking over other people's posts).[36]

Selfies, a social media form of self-portraiture, have become a powerful means for self-expression, encouraging users to share the most intimate and private moments of their lives—as well as engage in a form of creative self-fashioning, an embraced narcissism that turns navel gazing into high culture, and leisure-based consumption into a virtue.[37] This online behavior often mimics celebrities as a way to identify with idealized figures differently from parental figures that is typically seen in adolescent development. The fandom of Taylor Swift is 1 example of this type of embracement of media culture and idealized depictions of fame, talent, and beauty. It can be translated as a second form of separation-individuation from parental figures [for example, Blos, 1967].[38] Since one of the hallmarks of narcissistic behavior is a preoccupation with oneself and having a grandiose view of one's worth,[35] it is no wonder that our culture often describes those who frequently post selfies as exhibiting a public form of narcissism. On the flip side, a study of selfies made by Chinese college women found that posting selfies was related to positive self-esteem, wherein their social networks would provide positive feedback and enhanced body image which in turn affected their self-esteem.[39] More research is needed to understand whether those who tend to post selfies have high self-esteem and higher body esteem to begin with.

BODY IMAGE AND SOCIAL MEDIA SELF-CONSCIOUSNESS

Body image is a multifaceted construct that refers to perceptions of and attitudes toward one's own body.[40] Especially during adolescence, there is a heightened focus on appearance as individuals develop their physical identities. Since there is a societal focus on girls' physical appearance generally, girls tend to care more than boys about their online appearance. Over time, caring too much about your online appearance can lead to symptoms of depression.[41] "Imaginary audience" thinking is one of the developmental aspects of adolescence where they experience the sensation of being under a spotlight with peers as their audience. This social-cognitive phenomenon is likely intensified by the influence of social media and can affect body image. The current body of literature cautions about the emergence of a "perfect storm," where the features of social media (eg, idealized images of peers, quantifiable feedback), the developmental aspects of adolescence (eg, salience of peer relationships), and societal pressures (eg, societal over-emphasis on girls' and women's physical appearance) come together, possibly increasing the likelihood of body image concerns and related eating disorders.[41] For example, a study by Zheng and colleagues[42] of 963 female adolescents aged 12 to 16 year-old revealed selfie-posting on SNSs was positively associated with self-objectification, and this relation was moderated by imaginary audience ideation. Specifically, the influence of self-objectification on selfie-posting was stronger for young women with higher levels of imaginary audience ideation. An adolescent receiving a "like" on a post may not discern the specific reason—whether it is due to their appearance, other elements in the photo, the caption, or simply a gesture of support from a friend. In addition, a longitudinal study[43] found that appearance-oriented self-esteem was not significantly impacted when adolescents engaged in self-oriented social media use, such as curating their profiles and posting updates. In contrast, participants who engaged in other-oriented use, such as engaging with others' posts reported lower levels of self-esteem with regards to a particular form of self-esteem related to appearance. This relationship was stronger for female participants than males.

An explanation as to why some adolescents are more affected by body conscious-ness on social media than others can be found in self-worth contingency scenarios. Appearance-contingent self-worth is the degree to which one judges their own value and worth as a person based on their appearance and is positively associated with body shame, body surveillance, and negatively associated with appearance esteem.[44] Having a low level of appearance-contingent self-worth is protective, such that when confronted with any perceived threats to their appearance on social media, for instance, it is not as likely to threaten their own self-worth.[45] The degree of low versus high appearance self-worth is often dependent on a variety of factors including inter-sectional identity factors, such as race/ethnicity[46] and family support.[47] Additionally, adolescents who are in emotional distress may benefit from short-term interventions. Thai and colleagues[48] study found that reducing daily social media use has a short-term positive effect on body image among a vulnerable population of youth with emotional distress and heavy social media use. The 4-week intervention led to discernible improvements in both appearance and weight esteem compared to con-trol groups with unrestricted access to social media use.

The most popular social media (SM) sites for teens today are highly visual (eg, You-Tube, TikTok, Instagram). According to Objectification theory,[49] cultures that objec-tify bodies, socialize youth (especially girls) to believe that their physical appearance is of critical importance, often leading to self-objectification and body surveillance, which in turn lowers body esteem and increased depressive symptoms.[50] Subjec-tively, negative experiences on Instagram or Snapchat, in particular, impact body dissatisfaction through social comparison and body surveillance.[51] SM provides quantifiable feedback (eg, comments and likes) on public images, encouraging social comparison processes based on appearance, which can lead to appearance-related SM consciousness and poor body image. Girls have more appearance conscious-ness than boys and use more visually oriented social media platforms, such as Insta-gram, out of appearance related motivations and body image concerns compared to boys who are more likely to engage with gaming or less visually self-oriented plat-forms.[51] Also, visually oriented social media platforms may especially attract high self-esteem individuals to protect their already high self-worth, as they may expect to receive positive feedback in such a platform through likes or positive comments given its unique features.

Despite the vastly negative focus of research relating social media with body dissat-isfaction, the accepting nature of interactions with others on platforms can contribute to fostering positive self-esteem. Social media can also have a positive effect on body image by exposing users to more diverse representation and content. Body positivity challenges the unrealistic standards of beauty present in both traditional and social media by the promotion and acceptance of diverse body sizes and appearances.[52] In a recent micro-intervention study,[53] viewing body positive Facebook posts over a 2-week period improved body image and reduced women's appearance compari-sons. Viewing appearance neutral Facebook posts also improved women's body im-age. The micro-interventions had no impact on women's self-objectification. Body positive and/or appearance neutral posts may be effective micro-interventions for body image.[53] Therefore, individuals can find belonging and encounter people who resemble them on social media.

Theoretic and empirical work suggest that the body-positive movement may, iron-ically, lead to increased body image concerns among some young people, via exac-erbating the focus on physical appearance and increasing self-objectification. Ultimately, non-appearance focused media may be most promotive of body satisfac-tion. Consistent with this idea, "body-neutrality" (ie, appreciating a body's abilities rather than evaluating its appearance) has been identified as a potentially valuable avenue for addressing body image concerns and disordered eating among diverse adolescents (eg, gender-diverse populations).

CLINICAL VIGNETTES
This Case Vignette Illustrates the Beneficial Effects of Social Media in an Adolescent During a Severe Environmental and Social Traumatic Event

Sally is a 14 year old dedicated student and comes from a supportive and loving family. She had no prior psychiatric history. She has many friends, mostly girls and engages in friendships through social media and in person. Her self-esteem was stellar with good emotional connection with parents as well as being popular at school. During the coronavirus disease (COVID) pandemic she could not go to school or plan in-person activities with friends because her parents were very worried that she could get COVID and were controlling about what she could plan in person with friends. Over 6 months through the pandemic she became more isolated as it was difficult to coordinate activities with friends and even engage online with her school teachers and classmates due to non attendance. She felt progressively anxious and sad due to consistent isolation during the first months of the pandemic.

Sally has always been an emotionally intelligent individual and decided to spend most of her daily time online using Instagram, Snapchat, and Facebook to connect with her peers. She was able to develop good emotional connections with her friends that helped her to develop a sense of belonging to a group and continued to build her identity, relatedness and competence. She was asked to sign up for TikTok by her friends to share funny clips that would balance isolation and sadness of learning that people were getting sick and dying before the COVID vaccine was discovered. Sally built a solid social media profile for herself by posting pictures, comments, and jokes that allowed her to maintain relationships, help others, be expressive and meet new people. Later on when she felt that her self-esteem was coming back to her again with the same stability as before she was still engaged in social media but spending less time per day on it.

This Case Vignette Illustrates the Development of Isolation in a 13 year Old Boy with Social Anxiety and Low Self-Esteem

David is a 13 year old boy with social anxiety, Attention Deficit and Hyperactivity Disorder (ADHD) and persistent depression. His parents separated when he was 5 year old and his mother developed postpartum depression when he was born which impacted his attachment with her during his first year of life. He had very few friends and could not function well at school. He tried to compensate for his low self-esteem by being the class clown engaging at times in oppositional and defiant behaviors. David's father was absent and he lacked having a fatherly male figure with whom he could build on his identity. David spent many hours on YouTube looking into clips on how he could learn funny tricks in order to interact with others at school by continuing to be the class clown. He was developing a false self through hours of digging through YouTube and TikTok. As a result David was losing connection with classmates and did not make any friends but just acquaintances. He started to engage in the act of "lurking" keeping track of people online and also engaged in distracting thoughts such as social comparison with others. David became more lonely and depressed and started to question if life was worth living this way.

His pediatrician realized that David was developing a very negative self-esteem through social media and referred him to a psychiatric provider that started him on medication for his ADHD, anxiety and depression together with psychotherapy. After some time in treatment David stopped looking into how to be a class clown on You-Tube. Even though he was inattentive and impulsive at school, he spent very long periods of time engaged in social media. There was also a difference seen within his unstable "offline" self-esteem becoming more positive while engaging with other social media platforms such as WhatsApp, Instagram, and Snapchat. His classmates started to interact more with him, increasing his self-esteem and consequently lowering his anxiety, depression, and loneliness. He began to post pictures and interact with 1 or 2 real friends, building somehow a sense of belonging to an adolescent group.

This Case Vignette Illustrates the Dynamics of Selfies Toward the Discovery of Adolescent Identification with an Ideal Self Through Healthy Narcissistic Drives

Mary is a 11 year old girl and physically older than her stated age. She lives with her parents that she considers "controlling and overwhelming" in pressuring her to excel in school and engage in sports. Mary is not a sports person but an artistic soul. She loves music and is a Taylor Swift fan. She listens to Taylor Swift's songs constantly and follows her on Instagram. She is able to connect online through other Taylor Swift fans by posting selfies of herself mimicking Taylor's gestures and postures. Mary is trying to build up a wishful identification with an ideal "celebrity" object in order to create a sense of adolescent identification and belonging with her peers. Her desire to have a more artistic identity rather than athletic helps her explore new ways of appreciating different body types online. Mary's self-expression through selfies allows her to share intimate ideals in a form of creative self-fashioning through a healthy grandiose narcissism, making her feel free to explore exciting versions of her future self. This initiates a second form of separation-individuation, a phase in which kids start to deviate from needing parental approval for exploring identity development in adolescence.

RECOMMENDATIONS FOR PEDIATRICIANS AND ADOLESCENT CLINICIANS

Psychoeducation with parents about guiding adolescents to practice making friends in person as well as in their digital worlds is a crucial component to social development throughout adolescence. It is important to note that adolescents often interact with their peers in real life *and* online, and using technology to interact with their peers is considered developmentally appropriate for adolescents according to the American Academy of Pediatrics.[54]

Given the mixed evidence of self-esteem being positively or negatively affected by social media use, clinicians should avoid blanket statements that social media is only good or bad for one's self-concept. Prior research has indicated that there are several person-specific considerations that may influence how much social media use may impact self-concept, including personality, user motivations, upward versus downward social comparisons, body esteem, and contingent self-worth. For instance, some adolescents may feel a heightened sense of loneliness due to passive social media use, however others, particularly those with vulnerable or marginalized identities, may use social media strategically to reduce social isolation and improve their sense of belonging and group self-esteem [Charmaraman 2021; 2024].[19,55] We recommend a curious and non-judgmental stance in exploring social media use, self presentation in online spaces and self-esteem. Understanding important intersectional identity factors for a particular youth (for example race/ethnicity, gender, sexuality, etc.), the reasons behind social media use and how the young person feels about their social media use are helpful to explore.

In order to gain a better understanding of social interactions and behaviors online, clinicians might review how their patients use social media and identify areas for adjustment, such as pointing out a preponderance of upward social comparisons in hopes of reducing feelings of envy. In some cases, upward social comparisons can be beneficial, such that comparing oneself upwards on SNSs and engaging in positive self-comparison can lead to positive outcomes, such as feeling inspired, which are closely linked to well-being. For youth who identify ambivalence or negative effects on self-esteem related to social media use, using motivational interviewing techniques to identify possible behavior changes can be beneficial. For example, youth feeling badly after excessive upward self-comparisons, may take a break from the app, or start a new profile which effectively restarts the algorithm of generated content sent to them. Clinicians can help youth challenge cultural stereotypes about beauty, bodies and self-worth, encourage the development of healthy relationships in online and offline spaces and help youth develop healthy social media habits and behaviors.

Finally, due to the cross-sectional nature of most research linking self-esteem with social media, we need further research to understand the directionality of the influence. For instance, individuals may come to social media with pre-existing vulnerabilities regarding contingent self-worth or social media may exacerbate these vulnerabilities.[51]

CLINICS CARE POINTS

- All mental health evaluations of young children should include an assessment of the child's relationship with at least one primary caregiverWhen talking to adolescents clients, watch out for making any assumptions about their social media use. Ask questions about motivations and what they get out of social media - does the content fuel their low self-esteem or can it help to boost self-esteem?

- Parents could be advised to have not just one big media use discussion but to have these conversations early and often, in order to understand short-term and long-term impacts on self-esteem as they navigate the world of social media in the early adolescent years.

ACKNOWLEDGMENTS

The authors wish to thank the Class of '67 Internship Program at the Wellesley Centers for Women for funding to support the third and fourth authors. We are grateful to our editor Erin L. Belfort for valuable feedback on a previous version and to Vivian Huang for formatting assistance.

REFERENCES

1. Leary MR, Baumeister RF. The nature and function of self-esteem: Sociometer theory. In: Zanna MP, editor. Adv exp Soc Psychol, 32. San Diego, CA: Academic Press; 2000. p. 1–62. https://doi.org/10.1016/s0065-2601(00)80003-9.
2. Vogels E and Gelles-Watnick R. Teens and social media: key findings from Pew Research Center surveys. Pew Research Center, Available at: https://www.pewresearch.org/short-reads/2023/04/24/teens-and-social-media-key-findings-from-pew-research-center-surveys/, (Accessed 29 March 2024), 2023.
3. Rideout V, Peebles A, Mann S, et al. The Common Sense census: media use by tweens and teens, *Common Sense*, 2021, Available at: https://www.common

sensemedia.org/research/the-common-sense-census-media-use-by-tweens-and-teens-2021. (Accessed 29 March 2024).

4. Radesky J, Weeks H, Schaller A, et al. Constant companion: a week in the life of a young person's smartphone use, *Common Sense*, 2023. Available at: https://www.commonsensemedia.org/research/constant-companion-a-week-in-the-life-of-a-young-persons-smartphone-use. (Accessed 29 March 2024).

5. Nesi J, Mann S and Robb M. Teens and mental health: how girls really feel about social media, *Common Sense*, 2023. Available at: https://www.commonsensemedia.org/research/teens-and-mental-health-how-girls-really-feel-about-social-media. (Accessed 29 March 2024).

6. Rosenberg M. Society and the adolescent self-image. Princeton, NJ: Princeton University Press; 1965.

7. Parent N. Basic needs satisfaction through social media engagement: a developmental framework for understanding adolescent social media use. Hum Dev 2023;67(1):1–17.

8. Vogel E, Rose J, Roberts L, et al. Social comparison, social media, and self-esteem. Psychol Pop Media Cult 2014;3. https://doi.org/10.1037/ppm0000047.

9. Quatman T, Watson CM. Gender differences in adolescent self-esteem: an exploration of domains. J Genet Psychol 2001;162(1):93–117.

10. Williams ELD. The Impact of Team Sports on the Self-Esteem Development in Adolescent Girls. Dissertation. The Chicago School of Professional Psychology. 2023. Available at: https://ezproxy.wellesley.edu/login?url=https://www.proquest.com/dissertations-theses/impact-team-sports-on-self-esteem-development/docview/2817233067/se-2.

11. Guindon MH. Self-esteem across the lifespan: issues and interventions. Routledge; 2009. https://doi.org/10.4324/9780203884324.

12. Adams SK, Kuhn J, Rhodes J. Self-esteem changes in the middle school years: a study of ethnic and gender groups. RMLE Online 2006;29(6):1–9.

13. Mann RB, Blumberg F. Adolescents and social media: the effects of frequency of use, self-presentation, social comparison, and self esteem on possible self imagery. Acta Psychol 2022;228:103629.

14. Spies Shapiro LA, Margolin G. Growing up wired: social networking sites and adolescent psychosocial development. Clin Child Fam Psychol Rev 2014; 17(1):1–18.

15. Oyserman D, Fryberg SA. The possible selves of diverse adolescents: content and function across gender, race and national origin. In: Kerpelman J, Dunkel C, editors. Possible selves: theory, research, and applications. Hauppauge, NY: Nova Science Publishers; 2006. p. 17–39.

16. Balick A. The psychodynamics of social networking: connected-up instantaneous culture and the self. London, UK: Routledge; 2019.

17. Hunter A, Carlos M, Muniz FB, et al. Participation in a culturally grounded program strengthens cultural identity, self-esteem, and resilience in urban Indigenous adolescents. Am Indian Alsk Native Ment Health Res 2022;29(1):1–21.

18. Valkenburg P, Pouwels JL, Beyens I, et al. Adolescents' social media experiences and their self-esteem: a person-specific susceptibility perspective. Technol Mind Behav 2021;2(2). https://doi.org/10.1037/tmb0000037.

19. Charmaraman L. To connect or not to connect? That is the question. Cambridge, MA: Presented as part of *Social Media and Wellbeing in Context* at the Institute for Rebooting Social Media, Berkman Klein Center for Internet & Society; 2024.

20. Liu D, Baumeister R. Social networking online and personality of self-worth: a meta-analysis. J Res Pers 2016;64:79–89.

21. Mackson SB, Brochu PM, Schneider BA. Instagram: friend or foe? the application's association with psychological well-being. New Media Soc 2019;21(10): 2160–82.

22. Valkenburg PM, Koutamanis M, Vossen HGM. The concurrent and longitudinal relationships between adolescents' use of social network sites and their social self-esteem. Comput Human Behav 2017;76:35–41.

23. Nadkarni A, Hofmann SG. Why do people use Facebook? Pers Indiv Differ 2012; 52(3):243–9.

24. Charmaraman L, Grevet Delcourt C, Ben-Joseph E, et al. Social media and adolescent mental health. In: Halpern-Felsher B, editor. Encyclopedia of child and adolescent health. 1st edition. Amsterdam, the Netherlands: Elsevier; 2023. p. 337–50.

25. Ellison NB, Steinfield C, Lampe C. The benefits of Facebook "friends:" social capital and college students' use of online social network sites. J Comput-Mediat Commun 2007;12(4):1143–68.

26. Cacioppo JT, Cacioppo S. The growing problem of loneliness. Lancet 2018; 391(10119):426.

27. Pop LM, Iorga M, Iurcov R. Body-esteem, self-esteem and loneliness among social media young users. Int J Environ Res Publ Health 2022;19(9):5064.

28. Charmaraman L, Hernandez JM, Hodes R. Marginalized and understudied populations using digital media. In: Nesi J, Telzer EH, Prinstein MJ, editors. Handbook of adolescent digital media use and mental health. Cambridge, UK: Cambridge University Press; 2022. p. 188–215. https://doi.org/10.1017/9781108976237.

29. Cingel DP, Carter MC, Krause HV. Social media and self-esteem. Curr Opin Psychol 2022;45:101304.

30. Krause H-V, Baum K, Baumann A, et al. Unifying the detrimental and beneficial effects of social network site use on self-esteem: a systematic literature review. Media Psychol 2021;24(1):10–47.

31. Festinger L. A theory of social comparison processes. Hum Relat 1954;7(2): 117–40.

32. Bem DJ. Self-perception: an alternative interpretation of cognitive dissonance phenomena. Psychol Rev 1967;74(3):183–200.

33. Vitak J, Ellison N. "There's a network out there you might as well tap": exploring the benefits of and barriers to exchanging informational and support-based resources on Facebook. New Media Soc 2013;15:243–59.

34. Lopez RB, Polletta I. Regulating self-image on Instagram: links between social anxiety, Instagram contingent self-worth, and content control behaviors. Front Psychol 2021;12:711447.

35. Campbell W, Rudich E, Sedikides C. Narcissism, self-esteem, and the positivity of self-views: Two portraits of self-love. Pers Soc Psychol Bull 2022;28(3). https://doi.org/10.1177/0146167202286007.

36. Fegan RB, Bland AR. Social media use and vulnerable narcissism: The differential roles of oversensitivity and egocentricity. Int J Environ Res Publ Health 2021; 18(17):9172.

37. Murray D. Notes to self: the visual culture of selfies in the age of social media. Consump Mark Cult 2015;18(6):490–516.

38. Blos P. The second individuation process of adolescence. Psychoanal Stud Child 1967;22(1):162–86.

39. Wang Y, Wang X, Liu H, et al. Selfie posting and self-esteem among young adult women: a mediation model of positive feedback and body satisfaction. J Health Psychol 2020;25(2):161–72.

40. Cash TF, Fleming EC, Alindogan J, et al. Beyond body image as a trait: the development and validation of the Body Image States Scale. Eat Disord 2002;10(2): 103–13.
41. Choukas-Bradley S, Roberts SR, Maheux AJ, et al. The perfect storm: A developmental-sociocultural framework for the role of social media in adolescent girls' body image concerns and mental health. Clin Child Fam Psychol Rev 2022. https://doi.org/10.1007/s10567-022-00404-5.
42. Zheng D, Ni X li, jun Luo Y. Selfie posting on social networking sites and female adolescents' self-objectification: The moderating role of imaginary audience ideation. Sex Roles 2019;80(5–6):325–31.
43. Steinsbekk S, Wichstrøm L, Stenseng F, et al. The impact of social media use on appearance self-esteem from childhood to adolescence—A 3-wave community study. Comput Hum Behav 2021;114:106528.
44. Sanchez DT, Crocker J. How investment in gender ideals affects well-being: The role of external contingencies of self-worth. Psychol Women Q 2005;29:63–77.
45. Modica C. Facebook, body esteem, and body surveillance in adult women: The moderating role of self-compassion and appearance-contingent self-worth. Body Image 2019;29:17–30.
46. Dunn CE, Hood KB, Owens BD. Loving myself through thick and thin: Appearance contingent self-worth, gendered racial microaggressions and African American women's body appreciation. Body Image 2019;30:121–6.
47. Overstreet NM, Quinn DM. Contingencies of self-worth and appearance concerns: Do domains of self-worth matter? Psychol Women Q 2012;36:314–25.
48. Thai H, Davis C, Mahboob W, et al. Reducing social media use improves appearance and weight esteem in youth with emotional distress. Psychol Pop Media 2023;13. https://doi.org/10.1037/ppm0000460.
49. Katz E, Blumler JG, Gurevitch M. Utilization of communication by the individual. In: Blumler JG, Katz E, editors. The uses of mass communications: current perspectives on gratifications research. Sage; 1974. p. 19–32.
50. Choukas-Bradley S, Nesi J, Widman L, et al. The appearance-related social media consciousness scale: Development and validation with adolescents. Body Image 2020;33:164–74.
51. van Oosten JMF, Vandenbosch L, Peter J. Predicting the use of visually oriented social media: The role of psychological well-being, body image concerns and sought appearance gratifications. Comput Hum Behav 2023;144:107730.
52. Cwynar-Horta J. The commodification of the body positive movement on Instagram. Stream 2016;8(2):36–56.
53. Fardouly J, Slater A, Parnell J, et al. Can following body positive or appearance neutral Facebook pages improve young women's body image and mood? Testing novel social media micro-interventions. Body Image 2023;44:136–47.
54. Moreno MA, Radesky J. Putting forward a new narrative for adolescent media: the American Academy of Pediatrics Center of Excellence on Social Media and Youth Mental Health. J Adolesc Health 2023;73(2):227–9.
55. Charmaraman L, Hodes R, Richer AM. Young sexual minority adolescent experiences of self-expression and isolation on social media: A cross-sectional survey study. J Med Internet Res Ment Health 2021;8(9). https://doi.org/10.2196/26207.

The Impact of Social Media Use on the Development of Eating Disorders

Roslyn L. Gerwin, DO[a,b,]*, Sahar Ashraf, MD[c]

KEYWORDS

- social media • Eating disorders • Adolescents • Family • Advertising

KEY POINTS

- Critical thinking about social media content is an important skill for youth to develop.
- Some types of interactions and content exposure on social media, puts vulnerable youth at risk for developing eating disorders.
- There can also be positive online role models and communities for youth with eating disorders.
- Safe and healthy social media use among youth is dependent on education and monitoring by adults.

BACKGROUND

Eating disorders represent a heterogeneous cohort of illnesses across the lifespan. International ICD-11 and DSM-5 diagnostic classification tools recognize 6 principal clinical eating disorders (**Table 1**). A supplementary Other Specified Feeding and Eating Disorder category captures approximately 60% of cases that do not meet criteria for a more specific clinical diagnosis.[1]

This group of disorders significantly impacts psychosocial functioning and represents the highest mortality rate of any psychiatric disorder, other than opiate use.[2,3] The mortality rate of anorexia nervosa (AN), is 12 times higher than the mortality rate of all other causes of death for females 15 to 24 y old.[2] Twenty percent of people suffering from AN will prematurely die from physiologic complications related to their eating disorder.[3]

[a] Department of Child and Adolescent Psychiatry, Pediatric Psychiatry Consultation Service, Barbara Bush Children's Hospital, Maine Medical Center, 66 Bramhall Street, Portland, ME 04102, USA; [b] Tufts University School of Medicine, 145 Harrison Avenue, Boston, MA 02111, USA; [c] Department of Psychiatry, Texas Tech University Health Science Center, 2301 W Michigan Avenue, Midland, TX 79701, USA
* Corresponding author.
E-mail address: rlevine.gerwin@gmail.com

Pediatr Clin N Am 72 (2025) 203–212
https://doi.org/10.1016/j.pcl.2024.07.036
pediatric.theclinics.com
0031-3955/25/© 2024 Elsevier Inc. All rights reserved, including those for text and data mining, AI training, and similar technologies.

Table 1
Types of clinical and subclinical eating disorders and typical pathology

Clinical Eating Disorders	
Anorexia	An intense fear of weight gain and/or a disturbed body image that motivates severe dietary restriction or other weight loss behaviors
Bulimia	Recurrent episodes of binge eating and compensatory behaviors, for example, purging, to prevent weight gain
Binge eating disorder	Recurrent episodes of compulsive overeating that leads to distress without attempts to compensate for weight gain
Avoidant/restrictive food intake disorder	The avoidance or restrictive intake of food in the absence of body image concerns and fear of weight gain
Pica	Eating non-nutritive or non-food substances for a period of 1 month or more
Rumination disorder	Involves regurgitation of food after eating in the absence of nausea, involuntary retching, or disgust
Subclinical other specific feeding and eating disorders	
Orthorexia Nervosa	A pathologic fixation with healthy or 'clean' eating, avoidance of unhealthy foods and rigid dietary and exercise practices-violations of which cause severe emotional distress

Data from Alexandra Dane, Komal Bhatia. The social media diet: A scoping review to investigate the association between social media, body image and eating disorders amongst young people. PLOS Glob Public Health. 2023 Mar 22;3(3):e0001091.

For children and adolescents, the concerns are particularly relevant given that eating disorders represent the third most common chronic health condition and the prevalence continues to rise. The National Eating Disorder Association reported that helpline call volume went up 70% to 80% at various points between 2012 and 2020.[4] The Centers for Disease Control and Prevention reported that weekly emergency department visits for eating disorders increased in 2020, and then continued to rise into 2022, with the overall proportion of visits for eating disorders among adolescent females doubling.[5]

So what is the cause? Eating disorders, themselves, are complex illnesses, influenced by biologic, psychologic, cultural, and environmental factors. Certainly, there was an initial temporal correlation to the coronavirus disease 2019 pandemic; however, the trend has persisted. Recent evidence has begun to suggest a correlation between social media use and the development of eating disorders. This would not be surprising, as media exposure has long been considered an environmental risk factor with regarding the development of disordered eating.[6] From print media to TV to movies, social media represents the contemporary version of visual triggers.

However, social media also has its own unique characteristics compared to traditional forms of media. Traditionally, media content was created by a small number of writers and producers and was received by a mass audience. On social media platforms; however, anyone can be a content creator and 'influencer'. The "social" aspect of available platforms provides a forum for a more concentrated gathering of people than previously possible. Additionally, social media communication is often through photos and videos, in addition to chats. This technology-facilitated peer interaction, which is inherently visual in nature allows for more body comparisons, behavioral instruction, and online eating disorder cultures. For people of all ages, this can negatively impact self-esteem, but may be even more problematic for youth, who are more susceptible to social pressures.

Who Is at Risk?

In the 1990s, studies demonstrated the increasing discrepancy between the ideal body image portrayed in media versus the actual body size of American and Canadian women.[6] A trend toward increasing thinness in publications such as PlayBoy and fashion models was correlated to an increase in real-life weight. According to research conducted by The National Center for Biotechnology Information,"media is a causal risk factor for the development of eating disorders and has a strong influence on a person's body dissatisfaction, eating patterns, and poor self-concept."[6]

However, many people, including youth, consume media and social media, without experiencing negative consequences. Social media alone cannot be the sole villain in this narrative. There is clearly a pre-existing vulnerability among youth who develop problematic social media use or who experience negative outcomes related to their use. Overall, the etiology of eating disorders is complex, with prevalence hypothesized

---

Box 1
Etiology of eating disorders

Biological Factors:
- Genetic Predisposition
- Gender
- Obsessive-compulsive traits
- Autism spectrum traits
- High BMI
- Early Puberty
- Perinatal environmental influences (such as premature birth)

Psychological Factors:
- Personality traits (rigidity and perfectionism)
- Negative emotionality
- Body image dissatisfaction
- Low self-esteem
- Appearance schemas (psychological structures involved in processing self-related appearance information)
- Trauma history

Social Factors:
- Social isolation
- Peers (bullying, teasing)
- Parental eating problems (modeling)
- Culture
- Media exposure
- Acculturation
- Middle-high socioeconomic status

Adapted from: Alexandra Dane, Komal Bhatia. The social media diet: A scoping review to investigate the association between social media, body image and eating disorders amongst young people. PLOS Glob Public Health. 2023 Mar 22;3(3):e0001091.

as a result of various biopsychosocial factors (**Box 1**).[1] Most eating disorders begin in adolescence. Natal females still represent the largest proportion of cases; however, there is a notable increase amongst males, athletes, those with obesity, and sexual and gender identity minorities.[1]

This article will explore the ways in which social media can interact with the aforementioned risk factors to contribute to the development of an eating disorder. We will also highlight positive uses of social media, as well as ways in which providers can facilitate developing healthy media habits among youth.

DISCUSSION
Perception of Body Image, Health, and Wellness

The "ideal" body image continues to evolve over time informed by cultural influences and ideas about desirability. For example, fuller-figured European women in the 1500s were physical representations of their husband's status and success, as they could afford a higher volume and quality of food. As thinner bodies became more idealized, there has also been more medical focus on weight and overall health, with various efforts to quantify potential omens for poor health and even early death, such as the body mass index (BMI). We have even created "Ideal Body Weights" and average targets for pediatric growth charts. Additionally, the media is constantly providing messages on the "best" formula for a healthy lifestyle, though this tends to be an ever changing rhetoric. With the impact of repeated exposure through social media, it is no wonder that there has been increasing focus on getting and staying "healthy" in the general population.

While social media can certainly be helpful in the spread of relevant information and guidance from reliable sources, the internet, of course, is largely unregulated, and therefore frequently inaccurate. Youth are tasked with processing available information and making decisions about the credibility and impact of the information, which is filtered through their own individual resilience and risk factors. Most of the available information is not intended to cause harm. There are ranges of applications, for example, that aim to support productive weight loss and acquiring better health, yet can exacerbate eating disordered behavior in vulnerable youth.[7] Developing critical thinking about media is now a necessary task of adolescent development; however, it is not always modeled and taught in the context of schools, families and in provider's offices.

Social Media and the Biology of Eating Disorder Psychopathology

Body image develops based on complex interactions between physiologic, cognitive, and sociocultural factors. This occurs in the context of the significant and dynamic physiologic changes, which occur during adolescence.[8,9] The repetitive opportunities in social media applications for self-comparison to images of online "ideals" can be risky for those vulnerable to developing eating disorders, and damaging to those with established, active diagnoses. However, another important question is how can we understand more about the process of cognitive distortions inherent in people with eating disorders and how they are affected by such intense visual stimuli?

Research has begun to explore the process of visual mapping in the brain, and its correlation to disordered eating.[10] There is still only an early understanding of the underlying biology, but it is showing potential clinical importance. For example, discrepancies between the person's receipt of body signals and their corresponding interpretation has long been hypothesized as a core characteristic of AN. There may also be potential primary dysfunctions of sensory encoding, and disrupted visual processing and parietal association networks.[10] This can manifest as perceptual inac-curacies of their current body, as well as between their current and their ideal body. These perceptual distortions lead to both distress and subsequent eating disorder be-haviors. The term "compensatory behaviors" is apt, as the person is quite literally attempting to compensate for the resulting negative emotions by changing their phys-ical appearance. The challenge, however, is that there may never be a weight or level of thinness that provides enough emotional relief, or what feels satisfactory is so se-vere it results in medical complications or even death.

How this is affected by social media exposure is still poorly understood, but it is hy-pothesized that the repetitive exposure to visual content representing unhealthy body ideals (which is not present in other types of media the same degree) can trigger neurologic pathway abnormalities with higher frequency. Furthermore, there is a clear association between the frequency of comparing one's physical appearance to others on social media and the potential for body dissatisfaction.[11]

The Impact of Selfies

Studies have shown that adolescent uses of selfies can be indicative of a higher risk for developing an eating disorder.[12] In particular, the frequency and level of image manipulation prior to posting has had a measurable association with greater overvalu-ation of shape and weight, body dissatisfaction, and dietary restraint. Additionally, research has explored the direct psychologic impact of posting selfies, which can be negative.[13]

For many, posting a selfie on social media has either no consequences, or there is the positive subjective experience of immediate attention and gratification. This can occur even without image editing. However, some verbalize feeling increased anxiety, less self-confidence, and lowered mood after posting untouched photos.[13] It is impor-tant to caution against over-interpreting the impact of this effect. Even within this group, resulting negative emotions will be brief and have no longer term impact. This does represent a risk factor that can be monitored for and discussed, especially for those youth more prone to body image distortions.

The Role of Influencers

"I couldn't stop comparing myself," is a frequent statement from teens those who increasingly turn to social media influencers as role models and for life advice. An "influencer" is defined as someone with a social media presence and enough followers to "influence" an audience for some particular purpose. Focus areas may include life-style choices such as eating, exercise, and achieving certain body type goals. For certain youth followers what starts as a casual hobby can quickly devolve into an obsession. There will often be initial small dietary changes, such as eliminating sweets and adding in more fruits and vegetables. This may be followed by what seems like a reasonable amount of exercise. They likely get positive and reinforcing feedback from friends, family, coaches, and even their primary care physician.

The messages portrayed by influencers, and celebrities, can be difficult for youth to identify as potentially harmful, as they are frequently under a "health and wellness" la-bel. For those with more developed critical thinking skills and more robust self-esteem, evaluating the merits of things like weight loss tea and appetite suppressant lollipops, may come more naturally. They may not be triggered by 'What I Eat in a Day' videos that show an influencer highlighting their daily meals, or exercise videos target-ing a specific body part deemed a "problem area." However, once someone begins searching and viewing particular content, most social media algorithms will work to further promote that content.[14] More vulnerable youth can experience repeated exposure, leading to internalization of unattainable goals, such as obtaining the "perfect body," despite the routine use of filters and editing tools by online influencers and celebrities.

Additionally, youth witness the positive reinforcement influencers get from their followers. A recent CNN article highlighted a teen's experience with Instagram.[15] A 14 year old athlete described wanting to excel at "clean eating" and have the "most fit body" possible. After her initial searches, her feed became automatically filled with body types that she would consider "ideal." They were accompanied by "likes" and positive comments, which further reinforced the drive for this perfect image. At the time of the interview, she stated "I wanted to be liked and loved like they were." She began posting her own photos, seeking similar positive online feedback; however, this was harder than she anticipated, and she often received negative comments, such as being called "fat." Ultimately, her eating habits fully evolved into a serious eating disorder with life-threatening medical complications.

It should be emphasized that this type of effect from social media is neither universal nor guaranteed. There are certainly many youth who would either filter out negative online comments or not seek out the validation. However, identifying those who are vulnerable often happens after the fact, further supporting pre-emptive open communication with youth identifying psychologic risk factors and developing healthy online habits.

Pro-Ana/Pro-Mia

Definitions:
- "Pro-Ana": Short for Pro-Anorexia
- "Pro-Mia": Short for Pro-Bulimia

These are slang terms, which promote restrictive eating and purging behaviors as socially acceptable 'lifestyle choices', rather than dangerous psychiatric illnesses.[16] Pro-Ana websites are known for content promoting eating habits and compensatory behaviors, which support the obsession with thinness and obscure the efforts from detection.[16] The visual aspects provide "Thinspo" or "thinspiration", which emerged in the early 2000's, and became known as a group of image ideals to strive for. Initially, it was primarily celebrities and models, but a selfie culture has since evolved.[17] A documentary series, *Thinspiration*, came out in 2012, which further explored the Pro-Ana community's relationship to photography and self-images. Pro-Mia websites function similarly to their Pro-Ana counterparts, with both minimizing and even outright denying the potentially devastating medical consequences of disordered eating.

Just like other forms of social media, the danger does not just lie with the passive existence of these sites. The goal is to attract new users and keep people engaged in what has become a very strong belief system, which is frequently hostile to outsiders. According to recent media reports, approaches are quite persuasive and interactive, with high utilization of videos, social networking, and organized tactics to promote the Pro-Ana lifestyle.[18] A 2015 article highlighted how some sites require "proof" that you are dedicated enough to your eating disorder to be part of their group.[19] Anorexia was written to have been called the "Goddess of Emaciation," an externalized entity requiring capitulation from group members.

Positive and negative feedback is given based on one's success following rigid, low calorie meal plans, engaging in compensatory behaviors, and even feeling the physiologic effects of starvation. Developmentally, for vulnerable youth craving social acceptance, identity formation, and validation, these sites can be particularly dangerous. Research studies demonstrate similar risks, showing that online discussion of behaviors, outcomes, and perceived benefits is highly influential.[20,21] They also emphasize the importance of broad education to schools, parents, providers, and so forth of monitoring youth use of social media and recognition of potentially problematic online behaviors in all settings.

Parental Monitoring and Controls

It is strongly recommended that the adults in a family system have an active awareness of how a child is using social media. There can often be a more limited focus on how much time is being spent online, but, in fact, the content consumption on social media is as, if not more, important.[22] There are a wide variety of tools to support developmentally appropriate monitoring, though concurrent discussions about healthy habits and safe use is also required. Any use of parental social media controls may also provide an opportunity for teaching about self-acceptance, self-regulation, and critical thinking about content. Helping youth determine valid health-promoting information versus misinformation and disinformation is a crucial skill to develop. Additionally, it is worth noting that social media does not have to be considered "problematic" for these conversations to be beneficial, and in fact may be even more effective when considered a routine part of growing up and part of ongoing discussions. Resources exist to support families in getting quality information about social media platforms and available monitoring options, as well as facilitating family discussion-

Common Sense: Parents Ultimate Guide to Parental Controls
Google Family Link
Apple Parental Controls
AAP Family Media Plan

The Preventative Impact of Teaching Media Literacy Skills

As stated earlier, critical thinking about media is not necessarily an inherent ability for youth, and is best assumed as a skill to be learned. The generally accepted definition of "media literacy" is the promotion of said independent critical thinking when consuming media. There has been a general interest in eating disorder prevention programs, including exploration of improved media literacy for those at risk for developing eating disorders. Originally, research targeted print and screen media, which remains the primary body of research, requiring extrapolation of results for similar effects with social media use. More recently, studies have begun to explore social media literacy, with results reassuringly demonstrating comparable benefits.[23,24]

It is widely accepted that the cognitive distortions and health-compromising behaviors associated with eating disorders deeply involve body image dissatisfaction, internalization of societal beauty standards, and drives for thinness, all of which media can exacerbate. Media literacy typically aims to support challenging published visual ideals and reducing eating disorder perceptions and symptoms. Interventions may include highlighting image manipulation that is frequently implemented in visual media.

Regarding the efficacy of such prevention programs, there have been several meta-analyses, all reporting positive benefit. A more detailed exploration however, did show that effect sizes were influenced by the prevention approach. Those that focused only on the internalization of body image from media, versus also including media literacy, were less effective. Additionally, dissonance-based prevention programs, as well as those targeting selective interventions were more beneficial. Regardless of the approach, no prevention programs displayed negative consequences.[25]

The Positives of Social Media and Eating Disorders

There are certainly ways in which social media can play a positive role in the treatment and recovery from eating disorders. For example, the National Association of Anorexia and Associated Eating Disorders provide access to online support groups and informational blogs. Additionally, "Pro-Recovery" communities have become more prevalent on mainstream social media platforms. Emerging literature highlights that though these online communities can also become a place of visual self-comparison, there can be more opportunities for this to be a beneficial experience.[26–29] Unlike other groups that are specific to certain eating disorders, such as AN, general recovery groups, house a variety of body types, and may also include a wider range of genders and ages. Additionally, there are opportunities for positive role models, as groups may include those more established in their recovery journey. It has been hypothesized that in the right online space, social media can serve to reduce the stigma of eating disorders, by encouraging open dialogue about personal struggles.

SUMMARY

Over the last decade, there has been a spike in use of social media by teenagers and adolescents. This correlates to an alarming rise in pediatric eating disorders, prompting more attention to the content being displayed online on social media. More efforts are required to understand the evolving innovations used by social media platforms and websites to attract and engage children and adolescents. Robust attempts should be made to educate providers, families, and patients to promote healthy media habits and reduce the potential for physical and psychologic harm. Youth are more at risk due to the impact of social media and exposure to unreliable health content at their developmental stage.

CLINICS CARE POINTS

- Social media use can increase the risk for developing an eating disorder.
- The risk is higher for already vulnerable youth.
- Early identification of those at higher risk is a key.
- Education and discussion about healthy media use can be protective.

DISCLOSURE

The authors have nothing to disclose.

REFERENCES

1. Dane A, Bhatia K. The social media diet: A scoping review to investigate the association between social media, body image and eating disorders amongst young people. PLOS Glob Public Health 2023;3(3):e0001091.
2. Matheson, Datta N. and Lock J., Psychiatric News, Available at: https://doi.org/10.1176/appi.pn.2023.02.2.16, (Accessed 10 December 2023). 2023.
3. S. C. D. o. M. Health, Available at: www.state.sc.us/dmh/anorexia/statistics.htm, (Accessed 10 December 2023). 2024.
4. Katella K. Yale Medicine, vol. 2024, Available at: https://www.yalemedicine.org/news/eating-disorders-pandemic, (Accessed 10 December 2023). 2021.

5. Radhakrishnan L, Leeb RT, Bitsko RH, et al. Pediatric emergency department visits associated with mental health conditions before and during the COVID-19 pandemic — United States, January 2019–January 2022. MMWR Morb Mortal Wkly Rep 2022;71:319–24.
6. Spettigue W, Henderson KA. Eating disorders and the role of the media. Can Child Adolesc Psychiatr Rev 2004;13(1):16–9.
7. Eikey EV. Effects of diet and fitness apps on eating disorder behaviours: qualitative study. BJPsych Open 2021;7(5):e176.
8. Irvine KR, McCarty K, McKenzie KJ, et al. Distorted body image influences body schema in individuals with negative bodily attitudes. Neuropsychologia 2019; 122:38–50.
9. Markey CN. Invited commentary: Why body image is important to adolescent development. J Youth Adolesc 2010;39:1387–91.
10. Ralph-Nearman C, Arevian AC, Moseman S, et al. Visual mapping of body image disturbance in anorexia nervosa reveals objective markers of illness severity. Sci Rep 2021;11:12262.
11. Jiotsa B, Naccache B, Duval M, et al. Social media use and body image disorders: association between frequency of comparing one's own physical appearance to that of people being followed on social media and body dissatisfaction and drive for thinness. Int J Environ Res Publ Health 2021;18(6):2880.
12. McLean SA, Paxton SJ, Wertheim EH, et al. Selfies and social media: relationships between self-image editing and photo-investment and body dissatisfaction and dietary restraint. J Eat Disord 2015;3(Suppl 1):O21.
13. Mills JS, Musto S, Williams L, et al. "Selfie" harm: Effects on mood and body image in young women. Body Image 2018;27:86–92.
14. Harriger J, Evans JA, Thompson JK, et al. The dangers of the rabbit hole: Reflections on social media as a portal into a distorted world of edited bodies and eating disorder risk and the role of algorithms. Body Image 2022;41:292–7.
15. Sidner S, and Jones J. CNN, Available at: https://www.cnn.com/2021/10/09/us/instagram-eating-disorders/index.html, (Accessed 10 December 2023). 2021.
16. A content analysis of thinspiration, fitspiration, and bonespiration imagery on social media (2017, September). Journal of Eating Disorders, Available at: https://jeatdisord.biomedcentral.com/articles/10.1186/s40337-017-0170-2. (Accessed 10 December 2023).
17. e-Ana and e-Mia: A Content Analysis of Pro–Eating Disorder Web Sites (2010, August). American Journal of Public Health, Available at: https://www.ncbi.nlm.nih.gov/pmc/articles/PMC2901299/. (Accessed 10 December 2023).
18. Reaves J. Anorexia goes high tech. Time Magazine. Available at: http://www.time.com/time/health/article/0,8599,169660,00.html. Accessed May 3, 2010.
19. Brenneisen N, Vice, Available at: https://www.vice.com/en/article/vdx7ex/i-spent-a-week-in-a-pro-ana-whatsapp-group-talking-to-the-goddess-of-emaciation-876, (Accessed 12 December 2023). 2015.
20. Mueller R, Psychology Today, Available at: https://www.psychologytoday.com/us/blog/talking-about-trauma/201508/pro-ana-websites-encourage-anorexia, (Accessed 12 December 2023). 2015.
21. Mento C, Silvestri MC, Muscatello MRA, et al. Psychological impact of pro-anorexia and pro-eating disorder websites on adolescent females: a systematic review. Int J Environ Res Public Health 2021;18(4):2186.
22. American Psychological Association, Available at: https://www.apa.org/topics/social-media-internet/social-media-parent-tips, (Accessed 12 December 2023). 2023.

23. Kurz M, Rosendahl J, Rodeck J, et al. School-based interventions improve body image and media literacy in youth: a systematic review and meta-analysis. J Primary Prevent 2022;43:5–23.

24. McLean SA, Wertheim EH, Masters J, et al. A pilot evaluation of a social media literacy intervention to reduce risk factors for eating disorders. Int J Eat Disord 2017;50:847–51.

25. Stice E, Marti CN, Shaw H, et al. Meta-analytic review of dissonance-based eating disorder prevention programs: Intervention, participant, and facilitator features that predict larger effects. Clin Psychol Rev 2019;70:91–107.

26. Au ES, Cosh SM. Social media and eating disorder recovery: An exploration of Instagram recovery community users and their reasons for engagement. Eat Behav 2022;46:101651.

27. Clark O, Lee MM, Jingree ML, et al. Weight stigma and social media: evidence and public health solutions. Front Nutr 2021;8:739056.

28. Koreshe E, Paxton S, Miskovic-Wheatley J, Bryant E, Le A, Maloney D, National Eating Disorder Research Consortium, Touyz S, Maguire S. Prevention and early intervention in eating disorders: findings from a rapid review. J Eat Disord 2023; 11(1):38.

29. Branley DB, Covey J. Pro-ana versus pro-recovery: a content analytic comparison of social media users' communication about eating disorders on twitter and tumblr. Front Psychol 2017;8:1356.

Social Media Contagion of High-Risk Behaviors in Youth

Meredith Gansner, MD[a],*, Casey Berson, MD[b], Zainub Javed, MD[b]

KEYWORDS

- Social media • Social contagion • Adolescent high-risk behavior

KEY POINTS

- Social media's unique features facilitate the rapid transmission of ideas and behaviors among users, particularly adolescent youth.
- Youth with a history of high-risk behavior may be at particular risk of being influenced by graphic content viewed via social media.
- Pediatric clinicians should regularly assess the social media content viewed by their patients at risk.

BACKGROUND

Teenagers in the United States spend up to 9 hours per day on screens,[1] and nearly 20% report "constant" use of social media.[2] The increasing amount of time youth are exposed to social media content has led to growing concerns about how these platforms influence adolescent behavior. To date, social media has been implicated in the "spread" of several high-risk behaviors among populations of youth, including substance use, non-suicidal self-injury, disordered eating, suicidal behavior, and violence.[3–7] The process by which beliefs or behaviors are transmitted via social media is commonly referred to as *social media contagion.*

Social media contagion is a recent phenomenon, but mass media has long been recognized as a driver of social contagion. Books, television shows, movies, and newspapers can all be held culpable for influencing the actions of large groups of individuals through their storytelling. However, while *social media contagion* represents a single subtype of media-driven contagion, it distinguishes itself in important ways. Social media platforms are especially efficient vectors for spreading "contagious" ideas and behaviors, and their rapid evolution has made them challenging to study.

[a] Department of Psychiatry, Boston Children's Hospital, 300 Longwood Avenue, Boston, MA 02115, USA; [b] Department of Psychiatry, Prisma Health/University of South Carolina, School of Medicine, Greenville, Greer, SC USA
* Corresponding author. 300 Longwood Avenue, Boston, MA 02115.
E-mail address: Meredith.Gansner@childrens.harvard.edu

Pediatr Clin N Am 72 (2025) 213–224
https://doi.org/10.1016/j.pcl.2024.07.037   **pediatric.theclinics.com**
0031-3955/25/© 2024 Elsevier Inc. All rights reserved, including those for text and data mining, AI training, and similar technologies.

Review papers evaluating social media contagion research are often focused on a specific high-risk behavior (eg, non-suicidal self-injury). This approach makes it difficult to appreciate the phenomenon of social media contagion as a whole, and obscures commonalities shared by various forms of social media contagion. The hypothesized mechanisms enabling social media-driven spread of diverse ideas and behaviors are often identical. Furthermore, the same types of media contagion recur with the rise of each new platform, differentiated only by unique risks associated with that new platform's functionality. For example, one should expect social media content that promotes disordered eating to appear on any new video-sharing platform, and the risks will be similar to those seen with pre-existing video-sharing platforms (eg, YouTube, TikTok).

Here, the authors review existing research on identified forms of social media contagion influencing high-risk behavior among youth, certain traits that may make some youth particularly susceptible to this phenomenon, and limitations to scientific understanding of social media contagion. The authors also provide the reader with a broader conceptualization of social media contagion. By comparing and contrasting social media contagion subtypes, and offering a theoretic framework for how social media specifically facilitates social contagion, this article will help pediatric clinicians adopt a singular, standardized approach to the prevention and management of social media contagion in clinical practice.

Why Is Social Media Such an Effective Vehicle for Social Contagion?

To best understand social media contagion, it is important to appreciate the unique aspects of social media that make these platforms more influential than traditional forms of media. For a contagion to be effective, it needs both access and opportunity; social media platforms not only create an environment optimal for social contagion, they also connect a vast network of susceptible viewers.

An optimal environment for transmission

Several mechanisms have been proposed as drivers of social contagion. *Social transmission* is perhaps the mechanism most similar to a "real" contagious process, and posits that exposure to specific content in and of itself can influence a person to entertain thoughts or engage in behaviors related to that content (eg, watching a video on YouTube about non-suicidal self-injury triggers a teenager to cut themselves).[8] Social transmission is thought to explain how behaviors like suicidality could spread via news reports or television shows. However, in most instances, content exposure alone is not enough to influence individual behavior; environmental factors that increase host susceptibility are important when considering whether or not a behavior will be imitated.

These other factors include perceived *descriptive norms,* practices perceived to be "acceptable" or commonplace within one's community, and *injunctive norms,* behaviors that an individual believes one "ought" to engage in based on peer expectations.[9–11] In other words, individuals are more likely to participate in behaviors they believe "everyone else is doing" or that are expected to gain peer approval. Social media platforms offer engaging multimedia content through text, images and videos, and use algorithms identifying and catering to individual viewer preferences, which results in an artificially narrow range of content exposure, insulating the viewer from exposure to multiple, contrasting opinions. Thus, social media can provide unlimited access to multimedia content featuring a particular ideology or behavior, and repeated viewings of like videos or posts reinforces that thought or behavior by giving teens the impression that "everyone else" is thinking and behaving that way.

Similarly, exclusive, tight-knit communities with diminished external influence have long been known to be hotspots of social contagion, as demonstrated by the well-documented tendency for non-suicidal self-injury to spread within insular environments like college campuses, prisons, and inpatient psychiatric units.[12] Social media platforms allow for the creation of smaller, independent digital communities, fertile breeding grounds for social contagion.

Widespread access to large social networks

Audience is also a critical component of social contagion, as an early example of suicide contagion demonstrates. The eighteenth century publication of Von Goethe's novel *The Sorrows of the Young Werther,* depicting a romanticized protagonist who died by suicide, was followed by a noted increase in suicides among the book's young audience. "The Werther effect"[13] refers to the potential of suicide portrayal in mass media to inspire real-life suicidal behavior. However, *The Sorrows of the Young Werther* is by no means the earliest depiction of glamorized suicide in the literature. Shakespeare's *Romeo and Juliet* predated Von Goethe's novel, and culminated in the suicides of its heartbroken protagonists. *Romeo and Juliet* might also have been expected to inspire suicide contagion, but it reached a much smaller audience because of widespread illiteracy of the era.

Social media platforms have the ability to immediately present a specific idea or behavior to a nearly limitless audience. Social media influencers constantly design content to connect with a wide audience and maintain engagement, and their most engaging material is selected via algorithm to reach the largest audience. Adolescents are intentionally targeted by content producers for profit; it is estimated that major social media platforms make billions of dollars annually through advertising to minors.[14] By refining a user-friendly interface that caters personalized content targeting adolescents' reward-driven neurocircuitry, social media companies excel at capturing and sustaining the attention of a vast audience of teenaged viewers.

DISCUSSION

Still in the process of identity formation, status-conscious adolescents are susceptible to internalizing and imitating "viral" social media trends. While frustrating for some parents, the majority of these trends are harmless, not appreciably different from prior youth-driven movements championing specific fashion brands, music artists, dance moves, or pastimes. However, even non-viral social media content can still inspire contagion. Adolescents whose online activities center around a singular community with homogenous beliefs will be subject to the same pressures (both perceived and real) compelling them to think or act in accordance. Many of the following high-risk forms of social media contagion are believed to spread via such like-minded online subcommunities.

Suicide

Suicide contagion is among the most well-documented forms of social contagion. A substantial body of evidence supports the Werther Effect and the role of mass media in spreading suicidality.[15] Those most susceptible to suicide contagion appear to be those who identify with the character or individual who espouses or dies by suicide, and "copycat" suicides tend to be most common in the first few weeks following suicide exposure.[15–18]

Like traditional media (eg, books, newspapers), social media content has been implicated in varying degrees of suicide contagion. For example, exposure to suicide-related content on online forums has been associated with subsequently increased suicidal ideation.[19] Exposure to content concerning a suicide cluster (ie, a series of 3 of more united suicide events in a common space and/or in a contiguous time frame) may confer additional risk. Youth without a history of suicidality who experience exposure to suicide cluster-related social media content *during* a suicide cluster are significantly more likely to endorse both suicidal ideation and suicide attempts.[20]

To understand why certain types of social media engagement might confer a greater contagion risk, it is helpful to consider additional research exploring the Werther Effect. While most forms of media have the potential to drive suicide contagion, not all suicide-related media content will. Stories that sensationalize or promote simplistic explanations of suicide, or those that depict suicide as a means of accomplishing a goal, seem more likely to inspire suicide contagion.[15,21] Based on related research, specific words and phrasing are recommended when reporting on suicides,[22] and adherence to suicide reporting guidelines has been shown to decrease incidence of suicide contagion.[15]

There exists no single agency responsible for monitoring the wording of suicide-related social media content, and the sheer amount of available media content makes effective monitoring challenging. Social media accounts affiliated with reputable news outlets are more likely to follow suicide reporting guidelines than the social media accounts of individuals. Social media users, typically motivated by the prospect of obtaining "likes" and "shares," may be incentivized to post suicide-related content in violation of suicide reporting guidelines. Unfortunately, the tendency for social media platforms to reward the posting of content more likely to inspire harmful contagion is not limited to suicidal behavior.

Non-Suicidal Self-Injury

Multiple studies have reviewed non-suicidal self-injury (NSSI)-related content on social media platforms and found hundreds of message boards and videos concerning NSSI which are unrestricted and easily accessible to teenagers[4,23–25] NSSI-related content exists on most social media platforms to varying degrees, as some platforms tolerate or feature more posts portraying NSSI graphically or in a positive manner.[26,27] Graphic images of self-injury may be especially likely to provoke copycat behavior.[28]

Adolescent and young adult females appear more likely to view and post NSSI-related social media content, for various reasons. Some youth seek peer validation or support in abstaining, while others use these forums to facilitate their self-injurious behavior (eg, by learning new methods of NSSI or ways to conceal it)[23–25,27] Despite its theoretical benefits, youth access to NSSI-related social media content should be monitored carefully. Engagement with this contentmay as easily trigger as quell self-injurious urges, depending upon characteristics of the viewer and content viewed. Social media platforms may actually incentivize continued self-injury. A systematic review of studies on NSSI-related Instagram content determined that posts featuring graphic NSSI imagery were more likely to receive online attention.[29] If this finding applies to other social media platforms, even youth who turn to these forums to avoid self-injury may as a consequence feel compelled to self-injure and post about it to obtain online peer support.

Violence and Extremist Ideology

Exposure to media violence, particularly exposure to actual interpersonal violence, has been associated with youth engagement in violent behavior.[6] While many factors predispose an individual to engage in violent behavior, increasing evidence has found social media may be among them. In-person social networks are capable of "spreading" violence locally (eg, shootings within a city),[30] but epidemiologic modeling shows that online social networks may do so faster and to a larger geographic distribution.[31] Organizations studying extremist groups have emphasized the growing role of social media platforms in extremist recruitment and organization.[32]

Research linking exposure to violent social media content and real-life violence is often unable to confirm the directionality of this relationship. Youth harboring extremist or violent ideology are inherently more likely to seek out online content that reaffirms their beliefs. However, engagement with violent content may indeed lead to acts of violence. Online forums dedicated to extremist ideology create insular *echo chambers,* spaces in which group members "echo" one another's opinions, reinforcing violent ideology and sheltering members from exposure to alternative viewpoints.[33] Such echo chambers effectively synthesize moral outrage, a factor in the development of extremism that has been linked to social media.[34,35] Perceived limits in accountability for online behavior also contributes to greater invisibility and dissociative anonymity and imagination, resulting in an "online disinhibition effect," the tendency for individuals to act out more aggressively in a digital setting.[36]

Research linking the adoption of extremist ideology to social media forums further supports a contagion effect. Engagement with extremist forums, and having one's posts positively reinforced by other group members, predicts further radicalization.[37] For example, the individual who perpetrated the 2022 mass shooting in Buffalo, New York, cited platforms 4chan and reddit as formative to his racist beliefs.[38]

Substance Use

Youth exposure to depictions of drug or alcohol use via television, movies, and video games correlates consistently with increased substance use.[39] This effect has led to video game and movie rating systems designed specifically to flag substance-related content. However, social media platforms are not subject to such content warnings, and drug and alcohol companies have found creative ways to circumvent restrictions on advertising substances to youth. For example, product placement for drugs or alcohol can occur within music videos, and young adults exposed to e-cigarette product placement within music videos are more likely to report e-cigarette use.[40] Music videos featuring such product placement can be shared easily via social media platforms without flagging as an advertisement.

Substance-related social media content frequently portrays drug use in a humorous or entertaining light. In their review of 73 studies, Rutherford and colleagues found that over 75% of substance-related content on social media depicts substance use positively.[41] Social media platforms also give youth a means to visualize the drug and alcohol use of their peers. Many youth report seeing videos of peers intoxicated online,[42] and admired celebrities and influencers sharing about their substance use. The relationship between youth exposure to cannabis and alcohol-related social media content and offline substance use is mediated through perceived descriptive and injunctive norms.[43] Youth whose peers appear engaged in substance use on Snapchat or Instagram are likely to consider drug use to be normal or even expected. The degree to which substance-related social media content *causes* youth substance use remains debatable, as youth already engaged in drug use are more likely to seek out substance-related content. However, as peer influence is a well-established factor driving adolescent substance use, the potential influence of online peers is likely considerable.

Self-Diagnosis

Over the last several years, social media has increasingly become a means for adolescents to learn about and self-diagnose medical and psychiatric conditions. Social media platforms provide answers to the health concerns of youth without the perceived inconveniences of professional appointments, and allow teenagers to connect with peers who have similar concerns and experiences, which can promise validation and a sense of belonging.

Unfortunately, mental health information posted on social media is typically unreliable. Research indicates that more than half of TikTok videos about attention deficit hyperactivity disorder contain inaccurate information.[44] Social media depictions of tic disorders not infrequently misrepresent these disorders by displaying rare aspects of these conditions (eg, coprophenomena) at a disproportionately high rate.[45] Medical professionals are also increasingly seeing young patients reporting symptoms which appear influenced by social media, as well as unreliable self-diagnoses ranging from dissociative identity disorder and autism spectrum disorder,[46] to functional tic-like behaviors.[47] Self-identification of such rare diagnoses appears more common in female-identifying youth, and youth with uncomfortable internalizing symptoms like anxiety and depression may prefer to identify with these rarer neuropsychiatric diagnoses.[48] While these self-diagnoses may help some youth make sense of distressing experiences andgrant access to peer approval, attention, or affiliation, they could also enable avoidant behavior due to perceived disability from a self-diagnosed illness.[46]

Body Image and Disordered Eating

Social comparison, the process by which a person determines their own self-worth by comparing themselves to others, is an everyday psychological process. What differentiates social media-related social comparison is the ability to carefully curate self-portrayal. On social media, youth risk unfairly comparing themselves to unrealistic, idealized images of peers. This is especially true as it relates to body image, because photo filters and artificial intelligence allow for flawless seemingly-real renderings of one's physical appearance online. Aggregate findings from 26 studies confirm a correlation between social media content exposure and body dissatisfaction.[49] Research suggests that adolescent females may be more susceptible to body image-related social comparison, and the degree to which a teen engages either with appearance-related online content or related self-comparison may predict negative body image.[50,51] Resulting negative body image or low self-esteem may even mediate the relationship between social media exposures and dietary changes, including disordered eating.[52] Extensive use of image-based (as opposed to text based) social media platforms, popular among teens, has also been linked to eating disorders (ED).[7]

Adolescents may struggle to differentiate online advice promoting "healthy dieting" from content promoting ED behavior, especially those already engaged in such behavior. For youth with disordered eating, pro-ED social media content has been implicated in maintaining the behavior and delaying recovery.[7] Like NSSI-promoting social media groups, pro-ED online communities allow individuals to share information on ways to continue disordered eating, and reports shared by individuals striving to achieve specific metrics of thinness can create a sense of competition among community members.[53] Social media companies' efforts to ban pro-ED content have been largely unsuccessful. Content creators evade censorship by using coded language for community names and/or hashtags associated with pro-ED messaging.[54] Similar to other forms of social media contagion, the extent to which to pro-ED social media content *causes* disordered eating is still unknown. Again, the relationship is likely bidirectional; youth already struggling with disordered eating are more likely seek out social media content related to dieting or body image, which further reinforces the maladaptive behavior.

Forms of Adaptive Social Media Contagion

If social media can inspire youth engagement in harmful behaviors like self-injury or disordered eating, it might also be used to promote protective ideas and behaviors. Few studies document beneficial social media contagion or the leveraging of social networks to spread certain healthy behaviors, but examples do exist.

A small body of research evidence supports the use of "social media contagion" to spread accurate health information, particularly in the field of sexual health.[55] Sexual practices, substance use, and eating habits are thought to be most susceptible to influence by social networks.[56] Public health-oriented social media campaigns could theoretically counteract negative effects of social media. Visually-appealing social media campaigns featuring adolescent influencers may be most likely to influence a wide youth audience.[57]

Additionally, many adolescents credit social media platforms for helping them understand and engage with issues important to them.[58] This is evident in youth-driven social justice movements like "Black Lives Matter" or "March for Our Lives." By compelling viewers to adopt and espouse the ideology behind these moments, exposure to social media activism could influence youth mobilization and engagement with social causes. This form of social contagion can assist in valuable connections with like-minded peers and even identity development for some teenagers.

Adaptive social media contagion could also encourage help-seeking behavior. The character Papageno in Mozart's opera "The Magic Flute" considers suicide, but decides against it after being offered alternatives. Storylines in which characters choose an alternative to suicide, or news outlets that offer helpful resources (eg, the suicide hotline number) alongside reports of suicide are thought to drive this protective "Papageno Effect," making exposed viewers less likely to attempt suicide.[59] A contemporary example of the Papageno Effect is the 2017 song "1-800-273-8255" by the artist Logic, which takes its title from the U.S. suicide hotline number. The song's popularity appears to have resulted in increased calls to the suicide hotline, potentially saving lives.[60]

Given their accessibility and influence, social media platforms could similarly disseminate information about alternatives to suicide and normalize the process of accessing psychiatric help for suicidal ideation and depression. Strategic social media content featuring adolescents who overcame depression and/or suicidal ideation might help to counter the plethora of social media content perpetuating suicide contagion. Such campaigns could prove especially critical for youth living in communities where mental health disorders and care are still highly stigmatized.

FUTURE CONSIDERATIONS

The research methodologies most commonly used to study adolescent social media contagion have inherent limitations. Studies performing comprehensive content analyses of social media platforms are unable to confirm whether visualization of certain social media content directly results in high-risk behavior; survey studies depend on accurate recollection of what social media content was encountered prior to engaging in a high-risk behavior. Longitudinal studies that capture both existing social media content and mental health impacts of content exposure would yield study results that are more clinically meaningful. Additionally, use of technologies like smartphone-based ecological momentary assessment has demonstrated promise in furthering scientific understanding of adolescent problematic internet use.[61,62] Similar studies using smartphone applications to passively capture data on social media use in conjunction with repeated surveys regarding high-risk behavior could clarify

---

Box 1

Clinics care points: Preventative guidance surrounding social media contagion

- Recommend creation and maintenance of a family media plan that specifically outlines what social media platforms/content are allowed, how social media use will be monitored, and anticipated consequences if rules are broken (eg, increased parental monitoring to social media use or restriction of use for X amount of time)

- Provide psychoeducation to patient and parents/guardians about how social media platforms use powerful tools to personalize content in order to keep the user engaged

- Encourage parents/guardians to maintain an open dialogue with their teen about healthy media choices, how to think critically about social media posts, and ways to verify content veracity/authenticity

- Advise parents/guardians to assess the diversity of their teen's social media activities (eg, Is the child engaged with an unhealthy online community?)

- For youth with a history of engaging in high-risk behaviors that have been connected to social media contagion, parents/guardians should be cautioned about the existence of social media content that could perpetuate the behaviors

---

the mechanisms by which social media contagion occurs and identify which youth are most susceptible.

Unfortunately, the lack of robust clinical studies on social media contagion leaves unresolved challenges for pediatric clinicians. Without validated and standardized screening tools to assess for social media contagion, many clinicians remain unaware of its possible contribution to their patients' symptoms or behaviors. Furthermore, it is not yet clear which patients require regular screening, nor what management strategies are most effective in managing this process. Collection of high-quality data on social media contagion would also help to guide development of these important clinical tools.

For those young patients suffering from mental health symptoms who spend a significant amount of time on social media, clinicians should ask what they have learned about their conditions via social media, and whether they have online peers who deal with similar problems or diagnoses. Adolescent patients may even be willing to share

---

Box 2

Clinics care points: Managing high-risk social media contagion in clinical practice

- Advise parents/guardians to establish a concrete plan for active monitoring of their child's social media use; this may include use of parental control applications that restrict or track a user's online activities in addition to direct observation.

- Many youth access high-risk social media content when looking for emotional support or desiring to learn more about a particular condition or behavior; encourage parents/guardians to help find more healthy ways for their child to access peer support or reliable health information.

- Strategize with your patient and their family about how to avoid encountering potentially triggering social media content. They can consider the following:
  A. Deleting specific, potentially triggering social media platforms or platforms with similar functionality (eg, image-focused platforms for youth with disordered eating)
  B. Disabling social media notifications
  C. Establishing alternative, accessible, non-digital coping skills for use in distressing situations where the teenager might previously have used social media (eg, after an argument, or when anxious).

---

their social media feeds with their clinicians, which can reveal a great deal about what type of content the youth engages in and whether it may be problematic from a mental health standpoint. Patients who are triggered to engage in risky behavior after viewing related social media posts should be encouraged to make changes in platform application or phone settings to eliminate such content from their feeds. If a clinician is able to determine that a high-risk behavior or affiliation with a psychiatric condition addresses the unmet needs of a teenage patient (eg, for affiliation or peer approval), they should help the patient and family to brainstorm healthier alternatives that could also address those needs (eg, afterschool activities, religious involvement).

SUMMARY

Based on our existing knowledge on social contagion and mounting observational studies combined with anecdotal reports, social media platforms are capable of powerfully influencing adolescent behavior. Results from multiple studies support a significant relationship between related social media content exposure and adolescent suicidality, non-suicidal self-injurious behavior, disordered eating, violence, substance use, and self-diagnosis. However, convincing research evidence that social media exposures *cause* these behaviors is not yet available. As researchers continue to improve upon scientific understanding of this phenomenon, all pediatric clinicians should be aware of the potential of social media contagion to perpetuate or maintain maladaptive high-risk behaviors. Psychoeducation on social media contagion should be provided to pediatric patients and their guardians prior to the child's first independent social media use (**Box 1**). Most forms of high-risk social media contagion spread via similar mechanisms, and exist on multiple platforms, so a common standardized approach to clinical management of social media contagion is recommended (**Box 2**).

DISCLOSURE

The authors have nothing to disclose.

REFERENCES

1. American Academy of Child and Adolescent Psychiatry. Screen time and children. 2020. Available at: https://www.aacap.org/AACAP/Families_and_Youth/Facts_for_Families/FFF-Guide/Children-And-Watching-TV-054.aspx.
2. Anderson M, Faverio M, Gottfried J. Teens, social media and technology 2023. Washington, DC: Pew Res Cent; 2023.
3. Memon A, Sharma S, Mohite S, et al. The role of online social networking on deliberate self-harm and suicidality in adolescents: A systematized review of literature. Indian J Psychiatr 2018;60(4):384.
4. Lewis SP, Baker TG. The possible risks of self-injury web sites: a content analysis. Arch Suicide Res 2011;15(4):390–6.
5. Rutherford BN, Sun T, Johnson B, et al. Getting high for likes: exploring cannabis-related content on TikTok. Drug Alcohol Rev 2022;41(5):1119–25.
6. Ybarra ML, Diener-West M, Markow D, et al. Linkages between internet and other media violence with seriously violent behavior by youth. Pediatrics 2008;122(5):929–37.
7. Saul J, Rodgers RF, Saul M. Adolescent eating disorder risk and the social online world. Child Adolesc Psychiatr Clin N Am 2022;31(1):167–77.
8. Hawton K, Hill NTM, Gould M, et al. Clustering of suicides in children and adolescents. Lancet Child Adolesc Health 2020;4(1):58–67.

9. Bandura A. Social foundations of thought and action: a social cognitive theory. Prentice-Hall, Englewood Cliffs, NJ, USA.; 1986.

10. Masur PK, DiFranzo D, Bazarova NN. Behavioral contagion on social media: Effects of social norms, design interventions, and critical media literacy on self-disclosure. In: Smith J, editor. PLoS One 2021;16(7):e0254670.

11. Cialdini RB, Reno RR, Kallgren CA. A focus theory of normative conduct: recycling the concept of norms to reduce littering in public places. J Pers Soc Psychol 1998;58(6):1015–26.

12. Jarvi S, Jackson B, Swenson L, et al. The impact of social contagion on non-suicidal self-injury: a review of the literature. Arch Suicide Res 2013;17(1):1–19.

13. Jack B. Goethe's werther and its effects. Lancet Psychiatr 2014;1(1):18–9.

14. Raffoul A, Ward ZJ, Santoso M, et al. Social media platforms generate billions of dollars in revenue from U.S. youth: Findings from a simulated revenue model. In: Guidi B, editor. PLoS One 2023;18(12):e0295337.

15. Domaradzki J. The werther effect, the papageno effect or no effect? a literature review. Int J Environ Res Publ Health 2021;18(5):2396.

16. Fu K. Estimating the risk for suicide following the suicide deaths of 3 asian entertainment celebrities: a meta-analytic approach. J Clin Psychiatry 2009;70(6):869–78.

17. Park J, Choi N, Kim SJ, et al. The impact of celebrity suicide on subsequent suicide rates in the general population of Korea from 1990 to 2010. J Kor Med Sci 2016;31(4):598.

18. Stack S. The impact of the media on suicide. In: Shrivastava A, Kimbrell M, Lester D, editors. Suicide from a global perspective: psychosocial approaches. Hauppauge, NY, USA: Nova Science Publishers; 2012. p. 115–8.

19. Dunlop SM, More E, Romer D. Where do youth learn about suicides on the Internet, and what influence does this have on suicidal ideation?: Influence of the Internet on suicidal ideation. J Child Psychol Psychiatry 2011;52(10):1073–80.

20. Swedo EA, Beauregard JL, de Fijter S, et al. Associations between social media and suicidal behaviors during a youth suicide cluster in Ohio. J Adolesc Health 2021;68(2):308–16.

21. Phillips DP. The influence of suggestion on suicide: substantive and theoretical implications of the werther effect. Am Sociol Rev 1974;39(3):340.

22. American Foundation for Suicide Prevention. Safe reporting guidelines for media. Available at: https://afsp.org/safereporting/.

23. Whitlock JL, Powers JL, Eckenrode J. The virtual cutting edge: the internet and adolescent self-injury. Dev Psychol 2006;42(3):407–17.

24. Lewis SP, Seko Y. A double-edged sword: a review of benefits and risks of online nonsuicidal self-injury activities. J Clin Psychol 2016;72(3):249–62.

25. Brown RC, Fischer T, Goldwich AD, et al. #Cutting: non-suicidal self-injury (NSSI) on Instagram. Psychol Med 2018;48(2):337–46.

26. Picardo J, McKenzie SK, Collings S, et al. Suicide and self-harm content on Instagram: a systematic scoping review. In: Triberti S, editor. PLoS One 2020;15(9):e0238603.

27. Lewis SP, Heath NL, St Denis JM, et al. The scope of nonsuicidal self-injury on YouTube. PEDIATRICS 2011;127(3):e552–7.

28. Jacob N, Evans R, Scourfield J. The influence of online images on self-harm: a qualitative study of young people aged 16–24. J Adolesc 2017;60(1):140–7.

29. Miguel EM, Chou T, Golik A, et al. Examining the scope and patterns of deliberate self-injurious cutting content in popular social media. Depress Anxiety 2017; 34(9):786–93.
30. Green B, Horel T, Papachristos AV. Modeling contagion through social networks to explain and predict gunshot violence in Chicago, 2006 to 2014. JAMA Intern Med 2017;177(3):326.
31. Youngblood M. Extremist ideology as a complex contagion: the spread of far-right radicalization in the United States between 2005 and 2017. Humanit Soc Sci Commun 2020;7(1):49.
32. The Use of Social Media by United States Extremists. National consortium for the study of terrorism and responses to terrorism. 2018. Available at: https://www.start.umd.edu/pubs/START_PIRUS_UseOfSocialMediaByUSExtremists_ResearchBrief_July2018.pdf. Accessed July 3, 2023.
33. O'Hara K, Stevens D. Echo chambers and online radicalism: assessing the internet's complicity in violent extremism. Pol Internet 2015;7(4):401–22.
34. Crockett MJ. Moral outrage in the digital age. Nat Hum Behav 2017;1(11):769–71.
35. Neumann PR. Options and strategies for countering online radicalization in the United States. Stud Confl Terror 2013;36(6):431–59.
36. Suler J. The online disinhibition effect. Cyberpsychol Behav 2004;7(3):321–5.
37. Holt TJ, Chermak S, Freilich JD. An assessment of extremist groups use of web forums, social media, and technology to enculturate and radicalize individuals to violence. Washington, DC, USA: Office of Justice Programs' National Criminal Justice Reference Service; 2021.
38. Office of the New York State Attorney General Letitia James. Investigative report on the role of online platforms in the tragic mass shooting in Buffalo on May 14, 2022. 2022. Available at: https://ag.ny.gov/sites/default/files/buffaloshooting-onlineplatformsreport.pdf. Accessed February 6, 2024.
39. Jackson KM, Janssen T, Gabrielli J. Media/marketing influences on adolescent and young adult substance abuse. Curr Addict Rep 2018;5(2):146–57.
40. Majmundar A, Unger JB, Cruz TB, et al. Exposure to e-cigarette product placement in music videos is associated with vaping among young adults. Health Educ Behav 2022;49(4):639–46.
41. Rutherford BN, Lim CCW, Johnson B, et al. #Turnttrending: a systematic review of substance use portrayals on social media platforms. Addiction 2023;118(2): 206–17.
42. Morgan EM, Snelson C, Elison-Bowers P. Image and video disclosure of substance use on social media websites. Comput Hum Behav 2010;26(6):1405–11.
43. Cristello JV, Litt DM, Sutherland MT, et al. Subjective norms as a mediator between exposure to online alcohol and marijuana content and offline use among adolescents. Drug Alcohol Rev 2023;dar:13620.
44. Yeung A, Ng E, Abi-Jaoude E. TikTok and attention-deficit/hyperactivity disorder: a cross-sectional study of social media content quality. Can J Psychiatr 2022; 67(12):899–906.
45. Olvera C, Stebbins GT, Goetz CG, et al. TikTok tics: a pandemic within a pandemic. Mov Disord Clin Pract 2021;8(8):1200–5.
46. Weigle PE, Shafi RMA. Social media and youth mental health. Curr Psychiatr Rep 2024;26(1):1–8.
47. Frey J, Black KJ, Malaty IA. TikTok tourette's: are we witnessing a rise in functional tic-like behavior driven by adolescent social media use? Psychol Res Behav Manag 2022;15:3575–85.

48. Haltigan JD, Pringsheim TM, Rajkumar G. Social media as an incubator of personality and behavioral psychopathology: Symptom and disorder authenticity or psychosomatic social contagion? Compr Psychiatr 2023;121:152362.

49. Rounsefell K, Gibson S, McLean S, et al. Social media, body image and food choices in healthy young adults: A mixed methods systematic review. Nutr Diet 2020;77(1):19–40.

50. Revranche M, Biscond M, Husky MM. Investigating the relationship between social media use and body image among adolescents: A systematic review. Encephale 2022;48(2):206–18.

51. Jiotsa B, Naccache B, Duval M, et al. Social media use and body image disorders: association between frequency of comparing one's own physical appearance to that of people being followed on social media and body dissatisfaction and drive for thinness. Int J Environ Res Publ Health 2021;18(6):2880.

52. Blanchard L, Conway-Moore K, Aguiar A, et al. Associations between social media, adolescent mental health, and diet: A systematic review. Obes Rev 2023; 24(S2):e13631.

53. Lewis SP, Arbuthnott AE. Searching for thinspiration: the nature of internet searches for pro-eating disorder websites. Cyberpsychol, Behav Soc Netw 2012;15(4):200–4.

54. Gerrard Y. Beyond the hashtag: Circumventing content moderation on social media. New Media Soc 2018;20(12):4492–511.

55. García Del Castillo JA, García Del Castillo-López Á, Dias PC, et al. Social networks as tools for the prevention and promotion of health among youth. Psicol Reflexão Crítica 2020;33(1):13.

56. Smith KP, Christakis NA. Social networks and health. Annu Rev Sociol 2008;34(1): 405–29.

57. Chung A, Vieira D, Donley T, et al. Adolescent peer influence on eating behaviors via social media: scoping review. J Med Internet Res 2021;23(6):e19697.

58. Anderson M, Jiang J. Teens' social media habits and experiences. Washington, DC, USA: Pew Research Center; 2018.

59. Niederkrotenthaler T, Voracek M, Herberth A, et al. Role of media reports in completed and prevented suicide: Werther v. Papageno effects. Br J Psychiatry 2010;197(3):234–43.

60. Niederkrotenthaler T, Tran US, Gould M, et al. Association of Logic's hip hop song "1-800-273-8255" with lifeline calls and suicides in the United States: interrupted time series analysis. BMJ 2021;e067726. https://doi.org/10.1136/bmj-2021-067726.

61. Gansner M, Nisenson M, Carson N, et al. A pilot study using ecological momentary assessment via smartphone application to identify adolescent problematic internet use. Psychiatr Res 2020;293:113428.

62. Gansner M, Nisenson M, Lin V, et al. Piloting smartphone digital phenotyping to understand problematic internet use in an adolescent and young adult sample. Child Psychiatr Hum Dev 2022. https://doi.org/10.1007/s10578-022-01313-y.

Evidence-Based Evaluation of and Intervention for Adolescent Sexting

Elizabeth K. Englander, PhD[a],*, Paul E. Weigle, MD[b]

KEYWORDS

- Sexting • Cyberbullying • Depression • Anxiety • Case studies

KEY POINTS

- Sexting is not rare, but sexters are not a monolithic group. They sext for different reasons and motivations.
- Sexting because of negative pressure (eg, bullying, coercion) is associated with poorer mental health outcomes.
- Clinical approaches to different types of sexting behaviors should vary depending on risk factors present in each case.

INTRODUCTION

Responding to novel behaviors in a clinical setting is often difficult. In lieu of experience in evaluating poorly understood behaviors, judgments regarding the value and risks associated with these actions can be fraught with error. "Sexting," a term that refers to sharing naked pictures of oneself with another via digital media, can be particularly challenging to assess when presenting among children or adolescents.[1]

Sexting caught the attention of international media prior to the existence of substantial research evidence and was quickly associated in news stories with abuse and pathology.[2,3] Sensationalized sexting stories, combined with adult inexperience, lead many parents and practitioners to assume that any such behavior represents a serious psychological problem. The purpose of this article is to update practitioners on contemporary research regarding sexting and to help them identify cases involving high risk of harm compared to those which are more normative and less likely to involve negative outcomes.

[a] Massachusetts Aggression Reduction Center, Bridgewater State University, Bridgewater, MA 02325, USA; [b] Outpatient Services, Natchaug Hospital, 189 Storrs Road, Mansfield Center, CT 06250, USA
* Corresponding author.
E-mail address: ekenglander@gmail.com

Pediatr Clin N Am 72 (2025) 225–233
https://doi.org/10.1016/j.pcl.2024.08.006
0031-3955/25/© 2024 Elsevier Inc. All rights reserved, including those for text and data mining, AI training, and similar technologies.

pediatric.theclinics.com

BACKGROUND

Research on the frequency of sexting has produced a wide variety of results. A 2011 telephone poll by Mitchell and colleagues of a national sample of 1560 children and teens revealed variable rates, depending on the age of the respondent. Overall, only 2.5% of subjects reported making a nude image, and 7.1% reported receiving one during the previous year.[4] However, among 16 and 17 year individuals, rates of sexting were 31% and 41%, respectively. A 2012 study of sexting among 11 to 11 year old individuals, conducted by Dake and colleagues, found the same pattern, namely that while only 17% of all students engaged in sexting, 32% of 18 -year olds did so.[5] More recent research confirms that sexting among teens is neither rare nor universal: roughly half of youth reported having sent a sext before turning 19 years.[6] Older teens are substantially more likely than younger teens to endorse sexting, and rates of occurrence during extended time periods are higher still.

Several studies examined the association between sexting and mental health difficulties (eg, depression, anxiety). A study of older youth (18 years old) found no such association.[7] However, both age and context of the behavior have emerged as possible mediators of a link between sexting and psychopathology. One study of sixth graders found those who admitted to sexting also evidenced more depression.[8] Coercive sexting has been particularly associated with trauma and mental health symptoms.[9] Context surrounding sexting behaviors has emerged as key in understanding the possibility of a link between sexting behavior and psychopathology.[10]

TYPICAL AND ATYPICAL PRESENTATION OF SEXTING CASES

"Manuel loves me, that's what my mom doesn't understand!" insists Shyla, a 13 year old girl with a history of oppositional defiant disorder, major depressive disorder, and mild intellectual disability. Shyla struggles academically despite accommodations afforded by an individualized education plan at school. She feels rejected by most peers at school but has a few male acquaintances, and has recently refused to attend school more days than not. Her single mother works during the day, and Shyla is often home alone, entertaining herself via social media and video games and has made a few online friends. On a dating app, she met Manuel, a boy with whom she frequently discusses her depression and cutting habit, via text and video chat. Shyla recently learned that he is actually an adult and is married, but he reassures her that he plans to divorce his wife and marry her. He lives in a neighboring state and they have made plans to meet up in person.

When Shyla's mother discovered that she had sent him nude pictures via text, she confiscated Shyla's phone and forbade further contact. Shyla responded by telling her mother that Manuel is the only person who cares about her, and threatened to kill herself if her mother did not return her phone. Shyla's mother received numerous calls and texts from Manuel demanding to speak with Shyla to ensure her safety, and threatened to call DCF on her mother for neglect if she did not allow it.

A parent's worst nightmare, Shyla's situation constitutes sexual abuse and puts her at high risk of a host of negative outcomes. Similar situations have received a great deal of publicity through news stories, alerting parents and clinicians to the potential dangers of teen sexting. Parents frequently warn their children of just this type of outcome, implying that if they send naked pictures of themselves via text or social media, that it will be passed on and become public, will ruin their social reputation or college prospects, or even result in arrest for child pornography. Abusive situations like Shyla's serve as cautionary tales, but are they typical?

Let's consider the case of Cali:

"My daughter is a pervert!" exclaimed the mother of Cali, a 16 year old girl with a history of Attention Deficit Hyperactivity Disorder (ADHD), depression, and generalized anxiety disorder. Cali had been fairly high functioning for the past year with the support of weekly outpatient counseling, methylphenidate extended release, and escitalopram. During a routine follow-up, her mother expresses with great alarm that she looked through her daughter's phone after observing Cali acting strangely and spending excessive time in the bathroom. Her mother found nearly a dozen nude "selfies" which Cali had texted her long-term boyfriend Caleb, and vice versa. Cali's mother fears the pictures will be spread around to Caleb's friends and responds by confiscating Cali's phone and forbidding her from seeing him. She asks Cali's psychiatrist whether an inpatient admission would be appropriate to keep her daughter from dangerous sexual activity until she comes to her senses.

Cali is humiliated by her mother's response to her sexts. She relates that she and her boyfriend are not sexually active but she trusts him enough to send him the nude pictures over the last few months. She believes Caleb to be caring and responsible, which has been borne out by his actions and treatment of her. She feels that her behavior is not pathologic and hopes that her psychiatrist will convince her mother of this and help negotiate lifting her punishment.

Cali's mother is as concerned as Shyla's. Both girls engaged in sexting and both mothers are fearful of severe consequences. Are these fears equally justified?

RESEARCH EXAMINING SEXTING
Methodology

An anonymous survey examined 2252 youth during 2020, 2021, and 2022.[11] Subjects were aged 18 years and lived in Massachusetts, Colorado, or Virginia. They were never identified and knew the survey was confidential. Subjects were recruited to participate through the Subject Pool at 3 different universities, and most were required to engage in research as part of a Psychology course. The survey was approved by the Universities' Institutional Review Boards and administered online.

This study measured variables that are potentially useful in a clinical setting, including online sexualized behaviors such as sexting. Sexting, in this survey, was defined as sending a nude picture of oneself to a peer. The definition utilized did not include sexting via text (through messages or emails), or suggestive photos in which the subject was clothed.

Initiation and Frequency

Slightly more than half of all subjects (52%) reported having sent a nude photo of themselves. Almost three-quarters of these sexters (74%) indicated having first sexted before the age of 18 years, but more than half did not send a sext before the age of 16 years (61%). Around 19% sent their first nude picture at the age of 15 years, and another 19% sent it at the age of 14 years or younger.

Education about sexting was uncommon in this sample. Around 20% of subjects reported their parents had discussed sexting with them, while 23% stated that their parents had lectured them about the subject. Seventy percent of them stated that they had either received no education about sexting in school, or that the education they received made no impact on them.

Clinical implications

Sexting becomes more normative as youth age through adolescence. It is rare among pre-adolescents and uncommon among younger adolescents. Practitioners should not expect youth to have been educated by parents or schools about sexting.

OTHER CHARACTERISTICS OF SEXTERS

Both male and female participants engaged in sexting in this sample. Heterosexual females were more likely to report sending a sext compared to heterosexual males (56% vs 45%).

LGBTQ+ youth were more likely to report having sexted (true for male, female, and gender nonconforming subjects). This does not appear to be a consequence of different attitudes about sexting risk. LGBTQ+ subjects were no less likely to believe that sexting can lead to legal trouble, or that sexters can be harassed or bullied. They were, however, more likely to endorse positive views of sexting. For example, they were more likely to believe that sexting is a legitimate way to explore sexuality, that it can make people feel attractive, and that it is fun and exciting.

In this sample, 62 youth reported that they were either transitioning to another gender or were gender fluid or intersex. Among these youth, 60% reported sexting, which represents the highest rate of any group based on gender or sexuality.

UNDER WHAT CIRCUMSTANCES DO TEENS SEXT?

Most, but not all, teens sexted in the context of an ongoing relationship, as a way of exploring intimacy or sexuality. In this study, 67% of youth sexters sent the nude picture to a person they were dating (11% began dating the person after they sent the picture, and 56% were dating the person before they sent the picture).

Sexting was associated with sexual intercourse, in that youth who were sexually active were about twice as likely to report having sent a sext. However, it is notable that 66% of subjects reported having sexted before becoming sexually active.

Clinical Implications

Many sexters are dating, but they are not necessarily sexually active.

PEER PRESSURE

Many youth reported experiencing pressure or coercion to sext, but not all. Almost one-third (31%) of sexters reported no pressure at all. One-quarter (26%) of sexters experienced negative pressure, and another one-quarter (26%) experienced neutral or positive pressure. In this study, *positive pressure* was defined as pressure that was experienced as flattering attention or requests. Interestingly, 17% of sexters who were pressured, reported self-inflicted pressure to sext, namely, that they personally held certain beliefs that were central to their sexting behaviors (eg, believing their partner might break up with them, if they did not sext).

Most youth who reported pressure did not report that it was distressing for them, but almost all those who were very pressured (80%–90%) said that it was an upsetting experience.

Clinical Implications

Pressure by itself is not always indicative of a serious problem, but negative pressure or heavy pressure were experienced as noxious. Reports of pressure or coercion to sext—even self-pressure—should be carefully explored in a clinical setting.

IS SEXTING ASSOCIATED WITH MENTAL HEALTH CHALLENGES?

In this sample, sexters were more likely than non-sexters to report mental health challenges. For example, 62% of sexters indicated that they had experienced or were experiencing depression, compared to 43% of non-sexters. Similarly, 58% reported anxiety, compared to 45% of non-sexters. These differences were statistically significant. Sexters were also more likely to report problems with self-control and even self-injury.

Importantly, not all sexters were alike. In this sample, we were able to differentiate high-risk sexters (those who sext with strangers) from low-risk sexters (those who sext within an ongoing peer relationship). High-risk sexters were more likely to report anxiety or depression (69% and 72%). Differences between high-risk and low-risk sexters were particularly noteworthy when it came to problems with self-control (35% vs 22%) and, to a lesser extent, self-injury (26% vs 21%). Around 53% of high-risk sexters reported seeing a therapist or psychologist, compared to 36% of low-risk sexters.

Self-reported challenges with social skills and academic skills were unrelated to sexting, even among high-risk sexters.

The adolescent's age when sending their first sext was a significant mediator between sexting and psychopathology. As noted above, younger sexters have been found to be at greater risk for depression.[9] The current sample participants were all 18 years old, but they were asked the age at which they sent their first sext. Those who reported sending their first sext while in middle school were significantly more likely to endorse depression and self-injury, and somewhat more likely to report anxiety.

Coercive sexting has been particularly associated with trauma and mental health problems.[10] In this study, we hypothesized that sexting because of pressure, especially *negative* pressure, would be associated with mental health challenges. That hypothesis was robustly supported by the findings. For every mental health variable, negative-pressured sexters fared significantly worse than both positive-pressured sexters and non-sexters. For example, 77% of negative-pressured sexters reported challenges with anxiety, compared to 58% of positive-pressured sexters and 41% of non-sexters. Similarly, 79% of negative-pressured sexters reported depression, compared to 63% of positive-pressured sexters and 49% of non-sexters. The same patterns were observed for self-control problems, social skills, academic skills, and reports of self-injury.

Clinical Implications

Any sexting increases risk of mental health problems, but sexting in response to negative pressure or coercion is clearly more likely indicative of psychological dysfunction. Any youth who presents with sexting behaviors should be screened for mental health problems, but those whose sexting is a negative or even traumatic experience are significantly more likely to suffer mental illness.

CLINICAL EVALUATION

Available evidence supports screening for risky, traumatic, or negative sexting behaviors in patients whose clinical presentation suggests relevance. Younger teens with poor social skills, those who do most socializing online, those who have engaged in sexting and significant online conflicts in the past, those who spend more time unsupervised online, and those with poor decision making due to ADHD and particularly serious learning disabilities may be most likely to engage in high-risk or negative-pressured sexting, and clinicians should inquire about sexting behaviors in such cases.

At the same time, clinicians should withhold judgment about a patient's mental health status based *only* on sexting behaviors. Exploring concurrent risk factors, such as age of sexting onset, coercive peer pressure, and the context of sexting (eg, within an ongoing adolescent relationship) are key in determining psychological risk.

In Cali's case, some education helped improve the mother–daughter dynamic:

Cali's psychiatrist explains to her and her mother that sexting is neither rare nor deviant for today's adolescents. When done in the context of a stable, long-term romantic relationship it is not likely to result in negative outcomes, although those are still possible. Her mother appears dubious, but agrees to consider. Her mother calls the psychiatrist 1 week later to admit to having overreacted; she states, "thank you for talking me off the ledge and helping to put my daughter's behavior in a different light." She was able to have an open discussion with her daughter about the decision to engage in sexting with Caleb, express her concerns about the potential risk of harm to Cali. Ultimately, she returned her phone and expressed trust in Cali to make safe online decisions going forward. At the next appointment, Cali is grateful to her psychiatrist for mediating their conflict, happy that her mother accepts her actions and has reconsidered the related consequences.

PRACTICAL CONSIDERATIONS

Mental health clinicians are often reticent to ask our patients about sexting behaviors, even when it appears clinically appropriate. We fear making our patients uncomfortable, may be uncomfortable hearing details ourselves, or might feel judgmental about a patient's decisions to engage in sexting. Similarly, patients are often hesitant to share such experiences with their clinicians for similar reasons, often fearing being judged by the clinician, making the clinician uncomfortable, or having their confidential confessions reported to their parents. However, sexting experiences can sometimes have significant ramifications for mental health and safety, so it is clinically relevant to assess these behaviors in high-risk cases.

Assessing for sexting-related experiences should also be developmentally appropriate. For younger children at risk, it may be best to ask "has anyone online ever shown you something or asked you to do or show them something which made you feel uncomfortable?" For teens: "do you know what sexting means?" or "have you ever been asked to send naked pictures of yourself by someone online?"

When asking about sexting, it is also helpful to ensure that youth understand the boundaries of confidentiality. Clinicians can reassure patients by saying "I don't tell your parents what we talk about, unless you say it's OK or unless it sounds like someone might be really hurt if I don't." This may reassure youth who wish to share certain experiences with clinicians but not their parents.

Finally, it is often helpful to normalize sexting while asking patients about it. For example, a 12 year old girl with depression and self-harm reported to her clinician that she had become a pariah at school, her peers all teased her and rejected her ever since she and a boy in school broke off their romantic interests. This rejection hurt her deeply and drove her to cut herself, but she was vague about why her peers were teasing her. Her clinician neutrally explored the possibility of a negative sexting experience by commenting that "oftentimes girls send nude pictures to a boy they are interested in romantically, and sometimes the boy betrays their trust by passing on the pictures to others, which can be very embarrassing for the girl." The girl instantly responded, "that's what happened to me!" Framing sexting as a behavior that regularly occurs (even though it can be harmful) sends the message to our patients that we understand sexting can be normative and would not judge them for having engaged.

SUMMARY: WHEN DOES SEXTING INDICATE A PSYCHIATRIC EMERGENCY?

Many cases of adolescent sexting do not require clinical intervention. Teens who engage in low-risk sexting behavior may not require clinicians to intercede. It may be helpful for such youth to understand the difference between risky and less risky sexting. In cases where parents are worried about negative consequences that seem improbable, it may be helpful for clinicians to inform parents that such behavior is neither rare nor inherently pathologic.

In cases where a child or a teen is sending sexts in what appears to be a risky manner, it may be important for clinicians to explain to the child that while their behavior may be understandable, it can result in negative outcomes, including regret, embarrassment, or even the picture being passed on. It may be helpful for the clinician to problem solve with the youth what to do if and when such negative consequences arrive. Young people who have been exposed to pressure to send such pictures may be helped by problem solving with regard to how best to respond to this pressure, highlighting alternatives to complying.

In cases which involve an adolescent sending sexts to an individual significantly older or younger, it is important to assess whether this might constitute sexual abuse. When there is cause for concern, it falls upon the clinician to take steps to protect the child from further harm, regardless of whether the at risk child is a patient. This will typically include calling child protective services, but may also include informing the parent or even local police so they may take steps to protect the child from further harm. The clinician should inform the child that sexual pictures sent between a child or a adolescent and any significantly older individual is inappropriate, harmful, and often illegal. In such cases it may be helpful to problem-solve with the child on how to resist contact with the offender, and discuss with the child's caregivers how to prevent such contact. Close supervision of online activities may be warranted. Parental control software, such as that which comes built into devices such as iPhones, should be considered, but cannot completely replace traditional supervision. In serious cases, temporary confiscation of Internet-ready devices may be necessary. Parents have the option to replace a child's smartphone with a flip phone in cases where Internet access is deemed acutely unsafe but phone access is not. Parental supervision should be done in a manner which minimizes an adversarial relationship with their child whenever possible.

It is important for parents to understand that no method of restriction is foolproof. Motivated children may get a friend to lend them an Internet-ready device, sneak the use of devices when parents think they are sleeping, or find ways around parental control software, in order to contact the offender. However, efforts to prevent contact are often effective and should not be abandoned altogether.

Shyla's case was, unfortunately, one of these, and more significant interventions became necessary:

Shyla's psychiatrist expressed to her that her relationship with Manuel is inherently coercive and meeting him in person would risk assault. Shyla rejected these ideas and refused to speak any more about Manuel. The psychiatrist gathered information about Manuel from mother and contacted child protective services with a concern about child abuse perpetrated by Manuel, encouraging mother to do the same and to file charges with police. Mother followed the psychiatrist's advice to restrict Internet access, but Shyla responded by attacking her mother physically, leaving several bruises on her, and threatening to kill herself. Her mother, feeling unable to keep Shyla safe, called 211 which led to an emergency room visit and inpatient psychiatric admission.

Resources for Families

"Sexting and Relationships", a free online video which is appropriate for 8th grade and above, available at Commonsense Media at https://www.commonsense.org/education/digital-citizenship/lesson/sexting-and-relationships

American Academy of Child and Adolescent Psychiatry's Facts for Families regarding Sex: Talking to the Child, Social Media & Teens, and Sexual Abuse at https://www.aacap.org/AACAP/Families_and_Youth/Facts_for_Families/Layout/FFF_Guide-01.aspx#letterS

The Cyberbullying Research Center has a helpful summary of sexting research for appropriate for parents at https://cyberbullying.org/sexting-research-summary-2022.pdf

A description of how to use parental control software on iPhone and iPads can be found at https://support.apple.com/en-us/HT201304 and one for android devices at https://www.androidauthority.com/android-parental-controls-explained-3250229/

CLINICS CARE POINTS

- Physicians should screen for risky sexting behaviors among patients who are most likely to engage (eg, teens with poor social skills, those who do most of their socializing online, those who have engaged in online sexual behaviors in the past, those with a history of poor or impulsive decision making, and those with learning disorders).

- Screening for sexting may be most successful after a physician normalizes the act, asks in an age-appropriate manner, and reviews the boundaries of confidentiality.

- Parents of youth who sext should be reassured that sexting behavior can be normative and does not imply psychopathology.

- Adolescents considering or engaging in sexting should be warned of potential risks (the sext is shared without their consent, sender feels shame, suffers public embarrassment, blackmail, or rarely even legal consequences).

- Adolescents considering sexting should be advised never to sext to an adult or anyone they don't have an ongoing close, trusting, in-person relationship with.

- Any suspicion that an adult may be sending sexts to or requesting sexts from a minor should be reported to child protective services and/or police.

- Adolescents who have suffered negative consequences of sexting should be screened for related mental health problems including depression and social anxiety.

- Parents should be encouraged to talk to their latency- and teen-aged children about sexting, its risks, how the child can handle pressure to sext and what to do if they receive a sext.

DISCLOSURE

Both authors have no disclosures to make.

REFERENCES

1. Brown D, Sarah K. Sex, sexuality, sexting, and sex ed. Integrated Research Services 2009;76:12–7.
2. Dawson G. BBC newsbeat - 'revenge porn' is increasing in the UK, say charities. BBC Newsbeat 2014. Available at: http://www.bbc.co.uk/newsbeat/26851276.
3. Diaz K. Congressman Joe Barton, hit with 'sexting' revelation, bows out of 2018 race. Chron 2017. Available at: https://www.chron.com/politics/article/Congressman-Joe-Barton-hit-with-sexting-12395264.php.
4. Mitchell KJ, Finkelhor D, Jones LM, et al. Prevalence and characteristics of youth sexting: a national study. Pediatrics 2011;129(1):13–20.
5. Dake J, Price JH, Maziarz L, et al. Prevalence and correlates of sexting behavior in adolescents. Am J Sex Educ 2012;7(1):1–15.

6. Englander EK. Pornography, sexual activity, and sexting: LGBTQ youth. J Am Acad Child Adolesc Psychiatr 2023;62(10):S85.
7. Englander E. "Low risk associated with most teenage sexting: a study of 617 18-Year-Olds," research report, Massachusetts aggression reduction center. Bridgewater (MA): Bridgewater State University; 2012. Available at: http://webhost.bridgew.edu/marc/SEXTINGANDCOERCIONreport.pdf.
8. Chaudhary P, Peskin M, Temple JR, et al. Sexting and mental health: a school-based longitudinal study among youth in Texas. J Appl Res Child 2017;8(1).
9. Drouin M, Ross J, Tobin E. Sexting: a new, digital vehicle for intimate partner aggression? Comput Hum Behav 2015;50:197–204.
10. Englander E. Sexting, revenge pornography, and digital dating abuse: new research on adolescent digital behaviors. J Am Acad Child Adolesc Psychiatr 2016;55(10):S338.
11. Englander EK. Bullying and cyberbullying: what every educator and parent needs to know, second. Cambridge (MA): Harvard Education Press; 2023. Available at: https://hep.gse.harvard.edu/9781682538616/bullying-and-cyberbullying-second-edition/.

Digital Distractions and Misinformation

Kristopher Kaliebe, MD[a],*, Kaushal Shah, MD, MPH[b]

KEYWORDS

- Attention • Misinformation • Social media • Evolution
- Attention-deficit/hyperactivity disorder

KEY POINTS

- Digital opportunities for distraction have multiplied; thus, focusing on necessary tasks has become more difficult.
- Humans' social nature and bounded rationality create susceptibility toward environmentally influenced cognitive distortions such as groupthink and confirmation bias.
- Social media often distracts from productive activities and spreads misinformation; children and adolescents are uniquely susceptible to both.
- Attentional literacy is a multidimensional concept emphasizing the prudent use of personal attention resources via mindful awareness and thoughtful decisions.
- Clinicians can assess for attentional literacy and help families strategize to minimize goal interference and critically interpret online material.

INTRODUCTION

Over the past several decades, scholars have hypothesized that increasing exposure to media content endemic to our technologically-saturated world overwhelms the capacities of our primitive brains.[1–3] The exponential increase in available digital information has reached unprecedented dimensions. The amalgamation of the data from billions of individuals, as well as extensive business and governmental information repositories comprise the massive global datasphere projected to surpass 175 Zettabytes by 2025.[4] Herbert Simon's prescient insight from 5 decades ago resonates within this context: "What information consumes is rather obvious: it consumes the attention of its recipients. Hence, a wealth of information creates a poverty of attention and a need to allocate it efficiently."[1] Efficiently allocating attentional resources is increasingly critical in contemporary society's media-rich environment.

[a] Department of Psychiatry and Behavioral Neurosciences, University of South Florida, Tampa, FL 33613, USA; [b] Department of Psychiatry, Wake Forest University, Winston-Salem, NC, USA
* Corresponding author.
E-mail address: kkaliebe@usf.edu

Pediatr Clin N Am 72 (2025) 235–248
https://doi.org/10.1016/j.pcl.2024.08.002
0031-3955/25/© 2024 Elsevier Inc. All rights are reserved, including those for text and data mining, AI training, and similar technologies.

Children's and adolescents' cognitive faculties are immature, less able to grasp long-term consequences, and may be most at risk by this asymmetry between information and attention. Developing brains are more susceptible to distractions, including digital ones, which threaten to undermine their productivity and skill development. Educational pursuits are the most obvious casualty of digital distractions, especially as smartphone availability has proliferated and schoolwork is increasingly done via computers.[5,6] It is difficult for academic texts to compete with the stimulation these devices provide through platforms like social media. The presence of a smartphone can be particularly disruptive to cognitive tasks,[7,8] and seems to have a direct negative effect on academic performance.[9,10]

As ultra-social primates, children's and adolescents' attention is naturally drawn to culturally relevant and social information.[11] Youth copy or adapt behaviors they observe; and see themselves and the world differently when much of their experience and social life flows through the lens of social media. This is especially true for children and teens who typically spend most of their waking hours online.

Children and adolescents require guidance regarding how and where to devote their limited attentional reserve. Young people's attention is being pulled in more directions than ever, and there is a good reason for concern. Social media's influence on the enculturation of youth displaces the influences of parents, schools, and other societal forces. Rapid technologic advancements and financial incentives, along with the democratization, proliferation, and accessibility of social media content all facilitate this process.

Amid an intricate confluence of media and culture, Pegrum and colleagues introduced the concept of digital disarray.[12] Digital disarray refers to the combination of digital distraction with digital disorder (ie, the widespread circulation of online misinformation) and digital disconnection (ie, lack of engagement due in part to a negative view of the world and one's place in it), with eroded trust in online informations and institutions. Combined, these elements can produce disorientation and detachment from oneself and others.

Attentional literacy is a meta-concept[12] encompassing heightened self-awareness and honed focus. Attentional literacy draws inspiration from principles of mindfulness, advocating intentional awareness, and discouraging premature conclusions. By distancing individuals from reactive or habitual judgments, space is created for calm, rational analysis, and informed choices, enabling effective navigation of an environment rife with powerful distractions. Attentional literacy fosters a neutral, analytical, less biased approach to evaluate digital information. This concept emphasizes the need to manage our finite attentional resources and account for human irrationality. Parents and other caretakers can use the concept of attentional literacy as a lens to judge what guardrails will effectively protect youth from harm associated with social media and other distractions. Clinicians must respond to the need for attentional literacy by helping families effectively address digital distractions and related challenges.

HUMAN INFORMATION PROCESSING SYSTEMS

Human attention and information processing systems, integral to achievement, are susceptible to various limitations—processing speed, working memory, and sustainability.[13] Eric Charnov's "marginal value theorem," originally a theory in foraging biology, has been applied to information-seeking, highlighting digital behavioral patterns that echo animal foraging activities.[14]

Human sensory systems—sight, smell, taste, touch, and hearing—evolved to preferentially detect survival-critical cues in our environment. Prioritization of vital inputs means increased attention is paid to signs of danger, social conflict, sex, and food. Children learn to notice what others perceive as necessary, further guiding the direction of attention. Personal experience also strongly influences application of attention. The brain creates a coherent experience by ordering information from an array of sensory inputs.[15] Even during periods of directed focus (eg, during the act of reading), humans continue to monitor our environment, creating susceptibility to interruptions and distractions.

Smartphones, in particular, facilitate constant access to stimulating distractions.[9] Imagine a child attempting a challenging reading assignment. A notification appears as a flash on the screen accompanied by a familiar vibration and sound. The student wonders what that notification could be and who it might be from. His spotlight of attention is no longer focused on his reading assignment.

Interruptions, such as this notification, disrupt the top-down processing of the assignment via bottom-up awareness of the smartphone notification.[16] Top-down refers to higher cortical areas of the brain directing focus whereas bottom-up represents the range of internal and external sensory input coming from the environment rather than directed by higher brain functions. Humans continuously manage bottom-up processing to discern whether each sensory input demands an immediate response.

Our broad lantern of attention scans our surroundings. However, environmental scanning comes at the cost of intermittently disrupting the spotlight of focus shining on the task at hand. In the case of the student, shifting focus to the incoming text disrupts the attention required to make progress on schoolwork. Switching to and from the primary task creates inefficiency as it drains cognitive resources, reducing accuracy, and productivity.

Humans have a limited ability to control the spotlight of our attention, especially in a distracting environment. One of the biggest distractions for contemporary youth comes from social media. The powerful pull of social media is not a revelation. Humans are social creatures. Our internal "sociometer" automatically processes and prioritizes status, fairness, and group affiliation, influencing our social interactions.[17] Status-conscious young people naturally wish to keep abreast of the interactions and interests of their peers, including trends in youth culture. They seek to both join with peers and demonstrate their individuality.

The percentage of youth aged 13 to 17 who engage in multiple social media interactions daily increased from 34% in 2012 to 70% in 2018.[18] This trend of increasing social media engagement has continued as of 2022, when 95% of 13 to 17 y olds reported using social media.[19] Youth interact with social media more frequently and for longer periods than ever before, so it is increasingly essential to understand how these experiences impact their minds and behaviors.

In one study, researchers observed that when studying, students with access to the internet maintained focus on an academic assignment for just 6 min before switching tasks to a high-tech distractor.[20] Task-switching comes with a high cost to efficiency and productivity, and parallels engagement with the brief, fast-paced videos featured on social media platforms popular with youth.

This quick repeated switching of focus is often called "multitasking." Rapid task switching leads to feelings of productivity, even though relatively little has been achieved. Moreover, research has shown multitasking and attention problems are highly interrelated, and suggest that media multitasking may progressively impair capacity to maintain attention, leading to greater use of multitasking in a vicious cycle.[21] Social media interactions are highly stimulating and appeal to humans social instincts, in contrast to goal-oriented tasks such as academic work, which require repeated practice of effortful focus.

Nomophobia, as the fear of being without a phone connection, is commonplace in today's youth. Young people have become so accustomed to easily accessible, fast-paced entertainment that 76% of Greek students aged 18 to 25 endorse moderate to severe nomophobia; 81% of the time these youth used their smartphones was for social media.[22] This research suggests young people are overly attached to technology, risking wide-scale disruption of focus, task completion, and learning.

Patterns of heavy smartphone use in 7th to 12th graders have been associated with poorer academic performance.[23] At one of the United States (US) universities, researchers demonstrated that one additional hour of daily smartphone usage lowered the current term grade point average by 0.15 points on average.[9] Academic problems result from a confluence of factors, but digital distraction appears to be a standout. In an analysis of 159 American high school students, findings suggested students were distracted during homework about 38% of the time, constituting an estimated 204 h per year of unintentionally engaging with distractions while attempting schoolwork.[24]

Rising numbers of people are reporting difficulty focusing. Attention-deficit/hyperactivity disorder (ADHD) diagnoses have become increasingly prevalent over recent decades alongside the growing influence of screen technology. The increased rates of ADHD likely relate to better recognition of neurocognitive deficits, greater knowledge about and trust in treatments, and decreased stigma surrounding the disorder. Yet increasing complaints of poor attention may also reflect a response at scale to the overuse of distracting technology that weakens youths' ability to focus.[25,26] Increased exposure to digital media has been correlated with attention problems, although the nature and magnitude of this association have been disputed.

There seems to be bi-directional interaction, whereas excessive social media and other screen exposure erodes focus, and those with difficulty sustaining attention are in turn, especially susceptible to excessive use of social media.[27,28] Regardless of the mechanism of distraction, youth can benefit from exercising attentional literacy during times of intended productivity. By bringing to conscious attention instances of distraction, individuals are empowered to redirect their spotlight of attention back to the task at hand.

ADHD has been linked to more frequent and problematic use of social media.[25] Problematic social media use is an enduring preoccupation with and inability to refrain from using social media. Problematic use interferes with school, social, and/or family functioning, and is explored in detail in this issue by Vidal and colleagues. The complexity of attention-related complaints in youth with high degrees of media exposure makes it difficult for clinicians to differentiate the degree that attention problems represent primary neurobiologic disorders from that which results from distracting environmental stimuli. The capacity of stimulant medication to facilitate more measured use of social media in individuals with ADHD is unknown, yet it seems plausible that improving core ADHD symptoms may moderate social media habits.

MISINFORMATION, TRIBALISM, AND THE ATTENTION ECONOMY

Most online information is accurate, but online misinformation and disinformation are increasingly prevalent. *Misinformation* is defined as inaccurate information that the producer believes is accurate. *Disinformation* is inaccurate information that the producer knows is false. Both are becoming commonplace, leading our current era to be labeled the "misinformation age."[29] This change is caused in part by economic factors combined with human tribalism, and the resultant thought bubbles or echo chambers of like-minded individuals insulated from differing opinions.

Regulating the information to which young people are exposed is a challenge dating back to ancient times. Plato, in his 375 BCE. Republic, advised that children should only be exposed to simple stories emphasizing civic and personal virtues.[30] Today, the task of controlling information exposure for children and adolescents is far more daunting amid the massive array of unfiltered, objectionable content delivered by the internet.

While Plato expressed concern regarding fictional stories, children are increasingly exposed to non-fiction material (eg, "the news"). This is of concern, as news stories have become increasingly negative over time.[31,32] Humans pay disproportionate attention to negative news due to our inherent negativity bias. Negative information stimulates a greater response from our defensive minds, making frightening or upsetting information especially impactful and memorable.[33] This suggests audiences are drawn to crimes, tragedies, and institutional failures more than stories of progress, peace, and success. Combined with a morbid news environment, negativity bias leaves news consumers, including children, not better informed but excessively informed about negative events.

Legacy media and news prior to the advent of the internet were governed by regulatory mechanisms to protect younger audiences (eg, ratings, time-of-day restrictions, and channel segregation). News reports always reflect the values and prejudices of broadcasters, but fact-based, impartial journalism was more esteemed in pre-internet years.[34] Few regulatory mechanisms exist to protect youth from inappropriate content online. These factors make excluding marketing, misinformation, and developmentally inappropriate content nearly impossible. Financial interests and advertising strongly influence which content children and adolescents are exposed to online, prioritizing engaging viewers over information quality. Conversely, credible civic- and health-minded organizations are not structured to maximize engagement and struggle to compete.[35]

The nature of information dissemination on social media compounds the issue of misinformation, as false news spreads faster than accurate news.[36] Young people need to be taught to discern the truth from misinformation and disinformation. Resistance to deception is greatest in those who recognize their vulnerability to persuasion and can discern intent to manipulate their opinion.[37]

A 2022 Reuters Digital Report showed that consumer trust in news has fallen in the US to 26%, the lowest of any country surveyed (p 15).[38] This report also found that younger audiences place less value on impartial journalism (p 19).

Today's adolescents, deeply engaged with social media, are exposed by algorithms to highly-curated news stories that reflect their interests, biases, and attitudes. This algorithm curation increases engagement but may have the secondary effect of reinforcing excessively negative opinions and tribal beliefs. These may increase distorted perceptions and undue confidence that there are no viable alternative viewpoints.[39] Compared to previous generations, today's youth express more distress about hearing facts or opinions they do not like.

Amplifying these concerns is the increase in *visual misinformation*, in the form of manipulated or mischaracterized photos, charts, and videos. The most popular social media posts for young people are pictures and videos, which are significantly more likely to receive engagement than text alone.[40] Posted videos or photos have an especially powerful potential to influence children and adolescents. Allan Paivio's dual coding theory posits that processing a combination of written and visual representations of an idea leads to better recall than written representation alone.[41] Visual content arouses emotions more powerfully than text, and can enhance persuasive impact.[42]

Images, misleading or not, are more likely to remain in individuals' minds and influence their beliefs. Recent findings regarding health misinformation[43] indicate that graphics draw more attention, are more easily recalled, and are a common source of health misinformation. Content creators using state-of-the-art software create fake videos and graphics which are increasingly realistic and liable to fool viewers. Deepfakes are a manipulation technique that allows any 2 identities to be swapped both in their facial image and voice.[44] New editing technologies like deepfakes can be used to create videos portraying any individual engaging in any activity, in a manner difficult to discern from reality.

Another aspect of visual misinformation is the systematic misrepresentation of the human body as depicted in social media. During human evolution and up until the widespread use of mirrors, a culture preoccupied with self-appearance was impossible. Contemporary youth culture values regularly taking and viewing self-directed photos called "selfies." The idealized, often augmented, and carefully curated photos posted on social media lead viewers to believe their peers are more attractive than they actually are, and feel worse about their own appearance in comparison. Low body satisfaction is, in turn, associated with the susceptibility to depression, anxiety, eating disorders, gender dysphoria, and body dysmorphic disorder.[45–48]

Social media thus drives focus on other people's physical appearance and self-consciousness about how one appears on social media. Exposure to a large quantity of idealized faces and bodies, that is, visual misinformation, and social media-curated over-valuing of appearance combine to create a "perfect storm" of stressors, especially for teen girls.[45]

For all these reasons, our "misinformation age" fosters distrust and uncertainty among youth. Misinformation and over-exposure to negative news and age-inappropriate topics can instill anxieties by emphasizing failures and danger, fostering mistrust in institutions.

DIGITAL DISARRAY

Digital disarray[12] is a state of heightened distraction, information overload, diminished institutional trust, and resulting disconnection from oneself and others thought to be prevalent among today's youth. This state stems partly from exposure to excessive information via highly distracted digital environments, which undermines logical, precise thinking.

Digital disarray is influenced by other societal trends, such as delayed parenting, smaller families, delayed age of adulthood, and social isolation. Youth now face increased rates of depression, anxiety, and self-harm, particularly among heavy social media users and those with worldviews emphasizing grievances such as social disparities.[49,50] Limiting social media use to 30 min per day for 3 weeks was found to decrease loneliness, anxiety, and fear of missing out in college students compared to controls.[51]

Social media functions to bring people together. However, its popularity has exacerbated political and cultural polarization,[39] likely through divisive rhetoric (eg, highly emotional language, us vs them demonization, sensationalism, and exaggerations of crisis or harm). In such contexts, where extreme and hostile voices are rewarded with attention and praise, the full range of perspectives (eg, reasonable moderates) is driven into silence. Similar dynamics occur with adolescents, who are increasingly pressured into displaying support for ideologic and political causes on social media.[52]

Within ideologically or identity-aligned communities, attacks on those outside the group tend to increase in-group status.[53] Thus, expressions of emotional narrow-minded reasoning trump humble inquiry or acknowledgment of value in other viewpoints.[54,55] Social media creates an ecology where endorsing misinformation is often rewarded with prestige.

Within institutions, this phenomenon has led to what Jonathan Haidt calls *structural stupidity*, in which identity, ideology, and tribalism degrade intellectual exchange. Even formerly trustworthy academic, government, and professional organizations can become purveyors of misinformation.[56] Structural stupidity can occur in schools at every level. When vital societal institutions are dysfunctional, their imprudent policies adversely affect children and contribute to a breakdown in trust across society.[57] Resultant mistrust in societal institutions, combined with constant distraction, fosters the disengagement characteristic of digital disarray.

Multifaceted Solutions

Teaching attentional literacy

Attentional literacy is crucial for today's youth to function in the face of overwhelming information.[12] It refers to the deliberate and skillful direction of attention while maintaining awareness and focus. Its conception drew inspiration from principles of mindfulness, advocating intentional awareness and discouraging premature judgments.

By distancing individuals from reactive or habitual judgments, space is created for emotional calm, contemplative analysis, and informed choices. This enables the successful application of attention in the face of powerful distractions. Attentional literacy instills an unbiased, neutral, analytical, basis for evaluating online information.

Attentional literacy requires a basic understanding of the dynamics of human cognition and employs strategies to safeguard limited mental resources. Cultivating attentional literacy in children requires families, schools, and other caretakers to promote habits and practices that protect limited cognitive resources. Older children can gradually exercise increased agency and independent decision-making regarding their attention.

Young people spend more and more time online for education, work, and leisure, increasing opportunities for distraction. An awareness of limited attentional resources supports intentional use of time, which for many will result in less time on social media. *Digital minimalism* endeavors to bolster personal autonomy and well-being via prudent and constrained online interactions.[58] Limiting social media to only selected devices, such as a single tablet or the computer, may reduce distraction and temptation to over-engage.

Attentional literacy utilizes techniques to maximize focus, reduce strain, and gradually build productivity skills. Setting timers to limit work into "chunks" is one common strategy. Short bouts of intensive exercise[59] and other "micro breaks" result in small but significant benefits in reducing fatigue, boosting vigor, and increasing overall performance.[60]

Teaching digital literacy

Effectively navigating social media and other online spaces demand critical thinking and problem-solving skills. Young people benefit from having the capability to assess and utilize data sets and to comprehend how algorithms shape online experiences. Skills to collect, create, transform, and safely use digital information are acquired gradually by school-age children.[61]

Schools can teach developmentally appropriate digital literacy skills via specifically designed curriculums or integration into existing lesson plans. Part of the curriculum should be devoted to identifying online misinformation. This would involve helping children to recognize their own vulnerability to persuasion, detect manipulative intentions, and understand how emotions can mislead reasoning.[62,63]

Cognitive reflection tests are simple questions which demonstrate humans' tendency to use mental shortcuts to arrive at answers. The experience of making errors in response to simple questions highlights the value of deliberate, thoughtful cognitive processes over impulsive, habitual thinking patterns.[64] Participating in a cognitive reflection test can help young people challenge the tendency to adopt on intuitive but incorrect assumptions.

Other techniques include prioritizing credible resources over more convenient ones (eg, popular social media posts). Young people benefit efforts to check multiple sources and assess for bias or financial influence. They should understand the difference between more reliable sources (eg, a scientific authority) and less reliable ones (a nonexpert influencer).

Today's youth must be taught to navigate online safety, relationships, and privacy. They should be aware that others may track their online behavior in order to manipulate or even harm them. Parents and other caretakers have always been responsible for keeping children physically safe. Some safety risks (eg, child predators) have migrated online, particularly in social media spaces.[65]

Teaching constructive disagreement

As digital citizens, children and adolescents must develop the skills needed to participate in free and open exchange of ideas. Novel approaches are required to help them engage in productive dialogues across diverse perspectives.

Constructive disagreement refers to a respectful, humble, productive manner of debating ideas, allowing for reasonable intellectual exchange.[66] Constructive disagreement is the functional opposite of acrimonious, tribal conflict often seen on social media. Constructive disagreement is characterized by respect for other opinions, polite language, an ethical approach to disputes, and criticizing ideas rather than the person espousing them. The cultures of science and medicine have long-held formal and informal rules to promote rigorous and respectful scholarly exchange. The principles of these longstanding traditions can prevent tribalism, increase the productive exchange of ideas, and combat misinformation.

Children and adolescents should be taught that certain group dynamics can inhibit free and open exchange and lead to self-censorship. As families, schools, and communities raise the next generation of social media participants, we should aim to instill a humble tone of online dialogue and openness to varied perspectives.

Children can be taught the principles of constructive disagreement as a core component of digital citizenship. Explicitly teaching these values and courteous language creates a standard for respectful engagement.

Similarly, the leadership of medical professional organizations, including the American Academy of Pediatrics and the American Academy of Child and Adolescent Psychiatry, should utilize principles of constructive disagreement to safeguard scholarly dialogue and prevent structural stupidity.

Recommendations. It has become imperative for parents and other caretakers to actively monitor children's environmental distractions and social media's influence on socialization. Our propensity to learn naturally and automatically from our environment endows us with inherited cultural wisdom, for millennia guiding us in foraging, identifying potable water sources, and safeguarding against threats. More than ever, allowing our youth unregulated access to developmentally inappropriate and distracting content across social media is potentially dangerous.

To respond to risks to youth posed by information overload, misinformation, and disinformation necessitates a comprehensive approach involving various stakeholders.

Table 1
Recommendations

Priority	Recommendations
Age Appropriate Electronic Engagement	1. Caregivers are entirely responsible for screen media exposures prior to age 7, assuming children have negligible ability to understand the risks and consequences of social media and other online content. 2. Caregivers can allow the progression of partial autonomy to screen media from ages 7–14, as the child demonstrates abilities to responsibly navigate online spaces. 3. Caregivers can allow youth autonomy to navigate online spaces independently by age 15–18 as adolescents demonstrate ability to handle social media safely. 4. Make technology less stimulating (eg, turn device settings to grayscale). If the technology is less stimulating for the child as they grow, the child will be better able to tolerate low stimulation, potentially improving focus long-term. 5. Set age restrictions on devices so only certain activities, applications, and websites may be accessed. 6. Set time restrictions on the device itself for specific applications and the device in general. 7. Promote study and sleep hygiene by creating phone free zones and times. Restrict studying and productivity in a space used for only that purpose. Disallow phones or tablets in the bedroom past a certain time. 8. Use a traditional alarm clock rather than a device with a screen to help keep screens from the bedroom.
Poor attention/Poor Academic Performance	1. Support family's and individual student's attentional literacy. 2. Change the environment to direct attention toward desired goals, such as school work and chores. 3. Reduce exposure to electronic stimulation like social media and videos. Multitasking and distractions inhibit learning. 4. Restrict child's exposure to screens, particularly media with quickly changing scenes and very short videos. Chronic exposure to highly stimulating and fast-paced content may degrade attention. 5. Explain and encourage mindfulness during technological engagement. Effortful practice helps build skills, even when using technology. 6. During homework and study time, prioritize the physical environment and routine. Remove unnecessary devices from the work environment. Restrict access to unproductive distractions by disabling notifications or removing phone from room. 7. Use brief physical activity breaks to restore focus and increase productivity. 8. Restrict access to electronics prior to sleep and until morning. 9. Set time restrictions on the device for specific applications and use in general. 10. Promote study hygiene via distraction-free zones, with certain spaces reserved only for studying and productivity.

(continued on next page)

Table 1 (continued)	
Priority	**Recommendations**
Misinformation Concerns; including visual misinformation	1. Assess patient's and family's culture regarding health, body image and social media. 2. Teach patients how visual information, including distorted selfies found on social media, are misinformation which can precipitate body image problems. 3. Encourage prioritizing health over physical appearance, discouraging excessive efforts to curate an online image. 4. Through mindful interaction with social media, identify and reduce interactions which amplify body dysmorphia. 5. Understand that social media promotes uncensored visual misinformation, exacerbated by powerful image-altering software. 6. Promote digital literacy through debunking tribal narratives and teach the value of rationality as an antidote for negative body image.

Institutions

- Schools can implement measures to enhance students' attentional literacy and critical thinking skills, emphasizing the ability to evaluate and verify information.
- Schools should consider removing phones from the classroom and limiting unnecessary screen devices from a teen's workspace.
- Schools should foster an environment conducive to respectful dialogue, encouraging open discussions, and exchanges of diverse perspectives to help counter the spread of misinformation and encourage critical analysis.
- Government, academic, and scientific institutions can use their neutrality and credibility to counter financial and tribal interests by promoting balanced information, building spaces for constructive disagreement, and supporting online protections for youth.
- Medical organizations should enact policies to ensure the production of trustworthy information via reforms that decrease group-think, increase open scholarly dialogue, and circumvent structural stupidity.[56]

Clinicians

The recommendations below are meant to aid in improving the priorities indicated (**Table 1**).

Treatment of psychiatric disorders, whether via psychotherapies, medications, or other approaches, can also help youth curtail unproductive or harmful social media use.

A multifaceted approach involving educational initiatives, structural reforms in information dissemination, and fostering critical thinking skills among individuals is essential to combating information overload and the proliferation of negativity and falsehoods. Attentional literacy offers a menu of solutions.

SUMMARY

The notion that technologies such as social media are harmless tools warrants skepticism due to our inherent distractibility, tribalism, irrationality, and negativity bias. Scientific data clearly demonstrate how social media distracts children and adolescents from important tasks, especially academics. Social media has a unique ability to enculturate and educate youth, for better or worse, and may disproportionately amplify tribal thinking, bias, and misinformation. For young people today, constant digital distractions are a fact of life to manage.

Pediatricians, mental health professionals, parents, and other caretakers must consider these challenges. We should adjust our approach and advice to help our youth minimize the negative impacts of social media on education, socialization, and other aspects of their lives. We must be mindful of the limits of human attention, our susceptibility to misinformation, and the need to prioritize and focus on critical tasks. Children and adolescents must attain attentional literacy to live productive, rewarding lives in this digital age.

CLINICS CARE POINTS

- A youth reporting academic problems or attention problems should prompt an assessment of the child's and caretakers' attentional literacy.
- Digital distractions and information overload often cause attention problems and academic underperformance.
- The solution to attention problems will most often require changes to habits and their environment, not a diagnosis and medications.
- Clinicians' advice regarding social media content should emphasize our common humanity and promote the acceptance of humans' universal susceptibility to tribalism, cognitive distortions, and confirmation bias.

ACKNOWLEDGMENTS

The author wishes to acknowledge that Eric Lee Kraitman contributed to the writing of this article. He is currently a medical student at Mercer University School of Medicine, Macon Georgia.

DISCLOSURE

None.

REFERENCES

1. Simon Herbert. Designing organizations for an information-rich world. In: Greenberger M, editor. Computers, communication, and the public interest. Baltimore, MD: The Johns Hopkins Press; 1971. p. 40–1.
2. Chen L, Nath R, Tang Z. Understanding the determinants of digital distraction: an automatic thinking behavior perspective. Comput Hum Behav 2020;104:106195.
3. Hanin ML. Theorizing digital distraction. Philosophy & Technology 2021;34(2): 395–406.
4. Reinsel D, Rydning J, Gantz JF. Worldwide global datasphere forecast, 2021–2025: the world keeps creating more data—now, what do we do with it all. Needam, MA: IDC Corporate USA; 2021.
5. Girela-Serrano BM, Spiers ADV, Ruotong L, et al. Impact of mobile phones and wireless devices use on children and adolescents' mental health: a systematic review. Eur Child Adolesc Psychiatry 2024;33(6):1621–51.
6. Amez S, Baert S. Smartphone use and academic performance: a literature review. Int J Educ Res 2020;103:101618.

7. Skowronek J, Seifert A, Lindberg S. The mere presence of a smartphone reduces basal attentional performance. Sci Rep 2023;13(1):9363.

8. Hartanto A, Lua VYQ, Kasturiratna KTAS, et al. The Effect of Mere Presence of Smartphone on Cognitive Functions: A Four-Level Meta-Analysis. Technol mind behav, 2024;5(1: Spring 2024). https://doi.org/10.1037/tmb0000123.

9. Sapci O, Elhai JD, Amialchuk A, et al. The relationship between Smartphone use and students academic performance. Learn Indiv Differ 2021;89:102035.

10. Türel YK, Dokumacı O. Use of media and technology, academic procrastination, and academic achievement in adolescence. Participatory Educational Research 2022;9(2):481–97.

11. Herrmann E, Tomasello M. Apes' and children's understanding of cooperative and competitive motives in a communicative situation. Dev Sci 2006;9(5):518–29.

12. Pegrum M, Palalas A. Attentional literacy as a new literacy: helping students deal with digital disarray. Can J Learn Technol 2021;47(2):5–8.

13. Frischkorn GT, Schubert AL, Hagemann D. Processing speed, working memory, and executive functions: independent or inter-related predictors of general intelligence. Intelligence 2019;75:95–110.

14. Richards D, Taylor M. A Comparison of learning gains when using a 2D simulation tool versus a 3D virtual world: an experiment to find the right representation involving the Marginal Value Theorem. Comput Educ 2015;86:157–71.

15. Drijvers L, Holler J. The multimodal facilitation effect in human communication. Psychon Bull Rev 2023 Apr;30(2):792–801.

16. Gazzaley A, Rosen LKD. The Distracted mind: Ancient Brains in a high-tech world. Cambridge, MA: MIT Press; 2016.

17. Leary MR, Tambor ES, Terdal SK, et al. Self-esteem as an interpersonal monitor: the sociometer hypothesis. J Pers Soc Psychol 1995;68(3):518.

18. Rideout V, Robb MB. Social media, social life: teens reveal their experiences. San Francisco, CA: Common Sense Media; 2018.

19. Vogels AE, Gelles-Watnick R, Massarat N. Teens, social media and technology 2022. Washington, DC: Pew Research Center; 2022.

20. Rosen LD, Carrier LM, Cheever NA. Facebook and texting made me do it: media-induced task-switching while studying. Comput Hum Behav 2013;29(3):948–58.

21. Baumgartner SE, van der Schuur WA, Lemmens JS, et al. The relationship between media multitasking and attention problems in adolescents: results of two longitudinal studies. Hum Commun Res 2018;44(1):3–30.

22. Vagka E, Gnardellis C, Lagiou A, et al. Prevalence and factors related to Nomophobia: arising issues among young adults. Eur J Investig Health Psychol Educ 2023;13(8):1467–76.

23. Domoff SE, Foley RP, Ferkel R. Addictive phone use and academic performance in adolescents. Hum Behav Emerg Technol 2020;2(1):33–8.

24. Mrazek AJ, Mrazek MD, Ortega JR, et al. Teenagers' smartphone use during homework: an analysis of beliefs and behaviors around digital multitasking. Educ Sci 2021;11(11):713.

25. Dekkers TJ, van Hoorn J. Understanding problematic social media use in adolescents with attention-deficit/hyperactivity disorder (ADHD): a narrative review and clinical recommendations. Brain Sci 2022;12(12):1625.

26. Boer M, Stevens G, Finkenauer C, et al. Attention deficit hyperactivity disorder-symptoms, social media use intensity, and social media use problems in adolescents: Investigating directionality. Child Dev 2020;91(4):e853–65.

27. Ra CK, Cho J, Stone MD, et al. Association of digital media use with subsequent symptoms of attention-deficit/hyperactivity disorder among adolescents. JAMA 2018;320(3):255–63.

28. Beyens I, Valkenburg PM, Piotrowski JT. Screen media use and ADHD-related behaviors: four decades of research. Proc Natl Acad Sci USA 2018;115(40): 9875–81.

29. O'Connor C, Weatherall JO. The misinformation age: how false beliefs spread. Washington, DC: Yale University Press; 2019.

30. Jowett B, editor. The republic of Plato. New Haven, CT: Clarendon press; 1888.

31. Pew Research on delclining news. Available at: https://www.pewresearch.org/short-reads/2023/11/28/audiences-are-declining-for-traditional-news-media-in-the-us-with-some-exceptions/. Accessed April 7, 2024.

32. Aljazera 2022. Available at: https://www.aljazeera.com/opinions/2022/11/27/bad-news-headlines-are-indeed-getting-more-negative-and-angrier. Accessed April 7, 2024.

33. Baumeister RF, Bratslavsky E, Finkenauer C, et al. Bad is stronger than good. Rev Gen Psychol 2001;5(4):323–70.

34. Esser F, Umbricht A. The evolution of objective and interpretative journalism in the Western press: comparing six news systems since the 1960s. J Mass Commun Q 2014;91(2):229–49.

35. Kington RS, Arnesen S, Chou WS, et al. Identifying Credible Sources of Health Information in Social Media: Principles and Attributes. NAM Perspect 2021; 2021. https://doi.org/10.31478/202107a.

36. Wang Y, McKee M, Torbica A, et al. Systematic literature review on the spread of health-related misinformation on social media. Soc Sci Med 2019;240:112552.

37. Peng W, Lim S, Meng J. Persuasive strategies in online health misinformation: a systematic review. Inf Commun Soc 2023;26(11):2131–48.

38. Reuters digital news report. 2022. Available at: https://reutersinstitute.politics.ox.ac.uk/sites/default/files/2022-06/Digital_News-Report_2022.pdf. Accessed April 7, 2024.

39. Kubin E, von Sikorski C. The role of (social) media in political polarization: a systematic review. Ann Int Commun Assoc 2021;45(3):188–206.

40. Li Y, Xie Y. Is a picture worth a thousand words? An empirical study of image content and social media engagement. J Market Res 2020;57(1):1–19.

41. Paivio A, Clark JM. Dual coding theory and education. Pathways to literacy achievement for high poverty children 2006;1:149–210.

42. Seo K. Meta-analysis on visual persuasion–does adding images to texts influence persuasion. Athens Journal of Mass Media and Communications 2020;6(3): 177–90.

43. Heley K, Gaysynsky A, King AJ. Missing the bigger picture: the need for more research on visual health misinformation. Sci Commun 2022;44(4):514–27.

44. Mahmud BU, Sharmin A. Deep insights of deepfake technology: a review. arXiv 2021. DUJASE Vol. 5(1 & 2) 13-23, 2020.

45. Choukas-Bradley S, Roberts SR, Maheux AJ, et al. The perfect storm: a developmental–sociocultural framework for the role of social media in adolescent girls' body image concerns and mental health. Clin Child Fam Psychol Rev 2022; 25(4):681–701.

46. Littman L. Parent reports of adolescents and young adults perceived to show signs of a rapid onset of gender dysphoria. PLoS One 2018;13(8):e0202330.

47. Korte A, Gille G. Wahlverwandtschaften? Trans-Identifizierung und Anorexia nervosa als maladaptive Lösungsversuche für Entwicklungskonflikte in der weiblichen Adoleszenz. Sexuologie 2023;30.
48. Laughter MR, Anderson JB, Maymone MB, et al. Psychology of aesthetics: beauty, social media, and body dysmorphic disorder. Clin Dermatol 2023;41(1):28–32.
49. Bock S, Schnabel L. Distressed Democrats and relaxed Republicans? Partisanship and mental health during the COVID-19 pandemic. PLoS One 2022;17(4): e0266562.
50. Gimbrone C, Bates LM, Prins SJ, et al. The politics of depression: diverging trends in internalizing symptoms among US adolescents by political beliefs. SSM-mental health 2022;2:100043.
51. Hunt MG, Marx R, Lipson C, et al. No more FOMO: limiting social media decreases loneliness and depression. J Soc Clin Psychol 2018;37(10):751–68.
52. James C, Cotnam-Kappel M. Doubtful dialogue: how youth navigate the draw (and drawbacks) of online political dialogue. Learn Media Technol 2020;45(2): 129–50.
53. Rathje S, Van Bavel JJ, Van Der Linden S. Out-group animosity drives engagement on social media. Proc Natl Acad Sci USA 2021;118(26):e2024292118.
54. Macy M, Deri S, Ruch A, et al. Opinion cascades and the unpredictability of partisan polarization. Sci Adv 2019;5(8):eaax0754.
55. Druckman JN, Klar S, Krupnikov Y, et al. How affective polarization shapes 'Americans' political beliefs: a study of response to the COVID-19 pandemic. Journal of Experimental Political Science 2021;8(3):223–34.
56. Haidt J. Why the past 10 years of American life have been uniquely stupid. Atlantic 2022;11:2022.
57. Brady HE, Kent TB. Fifty years of declining confidence & increasing polarization in trust in American institutions. Daedalus 2022;151(4):43–66.
58. Aylsworth T, Castro C. The Duty to Promote Digital Minimalism in Group Agents. In: Kantian Ethics and the Attention Economy. Cham: Palgrave Macmillan; 2024.
59. Wollseiffen P, Ghadiri A, Scholz A, et al. Short bouts of intensive exercise during the workday have a positive effect on neuro-cognitive performance. Stress Health 2016;32(5):514–23.
60. Albulescu P, Macsinga I, Rusu A, et al. "Give me a break!" A systematic review and meta-analysis on the efficacy of micro-breaks for increasing well-being and performance. PLoS One 2022;17(8):e0272460.
61. Lazonder AW, Walraven A, Gijlers H, et al. Longitudinal assessment of digital literacy in children: findings from a large Dutch single-school study. Comput Educ 2020;143:103681.
62. Van Der Linden S. Misinformation: susceptibility, spread, and interventions to immunize the public. Nat Med 2022;28(3):460–7.
63. Martel C, Pennycook G, Rand DG. Reliance on emotion promotes belief in fake news. Cogn Res Princ Implic 2020;5:1–20.
64. Toplak ME, West RF, Stanovich KE. The Cognitive Reflection Test as a predictor of performance on heuristics-and-biases tasks. Mem Cognit 2011;39(7):1275–89.
65. Ringenberg TR, Seigfried-Spellar KC, Rayz JM, et al. A scoping review of child grooming strategies: pre-and post-internet. Child Abuse Negl 2022;123:105392.
66. Sauer H. Can't we all disagree more constructively? Moral foundations, moral reasoning, and political disagreement. Neuroethics 2015;8:153–69.

Cracking the Algorithm
How to Ask the Right Questions about Social Media During the Interview

Fadi J. Hamati, MD[a], Jeremy A. Chapman, MD[b],*,
Ashvin Sood, MD[b]

KEYWORDS

- Social media • TikTok • Snapchat • Mental health • Instagram
- Psychiatric interview • Social media use • Passive–active use

KEY POINTS

- Social media use continues to evolve rapidly, yet efforts lag in evaluating its use and understanding its impact on adolescents.
- The authors propose a function-based framework that assists clinicians in identifying specific use patterns among adolescents.
- The authors guide readers through an algorithmic approach to implement the framework and assess for individualized risk and resilience profiles.

INTRODUCTION

Caleb, a 16 year old transgender male with a history of depression and gender dysphoria presents with his family for a follow-up visit. Exchanging greetings, you quickly notice that Caleb is glued to his phone screen, oblivious to the conversation going on. As he scrolls through intricately curated TikTok videos of chiseled jaws and sculpted bodies, a Snapchat notification opens to a 5 second transient image of his school friend, interrupting this stream of perfection. This scene has become a motif in this digital revolution as more and more teens gain instant access to the Internet through their smartphones.

It is almost impossible to find an adolescent without a smartphone. A 2023 survey conducted by Pew Research Center found that almost 95% of adolescents in the United States had access to a smartphone at home.[1] A Common Sense Media Census report showed that up to 88% of teenagers owned smartphones in 2021, compared to 67% in 2015.[2] With over 9 in 10 reporting daily Internet usage, adolescents in the

[a] Department of Psychiatry, Northwestern Memorial Hospital, Chicago, IL, USA; [b] Department of Psychiatry, SSM Health Treffert Center and Treffert Studios, WI, USA
* Corresponding author.
E-mail address: jeremy.chapman@ssmhealth.com

Pediatr Clin N Am 72 (2025) 249–265
https://doi.org/10.1016/j.pcl.2024.08.003 **pediatric.theclinics.com**
0031-3955/25/© 2024 Elsevier Inc. All rights reserved, including those for text and data mining, AI training, and similar technologies.

United States have been averaging 4.8 hours of screen time per day.[3] Unsurprisingly, the percentage of teens who are online "almost constantly" has nearly doubled since 2014 to 2015 from 24% to 46% in 2023.[1,3] This digital revolution contributed to the rapid rise and adoption of SM, especially among adolescents.[4] As you accompany Caleb to your office, you wonder to yourself: what are the implications of Caleb's social media (SM) use?

Adolescence represents a critical period of development during which teens acquire a sense of self and foster peer-relationships.[5] Many researchers have highlighted a possible link between this rise in SM use and the increase in prevalence of depression, anxiety, suicide, and risky behavior.[6,7] However, the strength of this association remains in question.[8] One thing is clear: SM is here to stay. Therefore, screening for SM use patterns in adolescents is essential to developing a more nuanced assessment of their mental health and well-being.[9]

The problem with evaluating SM use is that teens adopt platforms at a much more rapid pace compared to the development of research or clinical practice. The authors use "platform" to refer to any social media application or Web site such as Instagram or TikTok. Although the overarching trend shows a dramatic rise in SM use, a closer look at platform-specific preferences paints a more complex picture.[10] SM giants such as MySpace and Friendster have been replaced by emerging players such as TikTok and Instagram.[10] These new platforms influence online trends and shape real-life narratives, especially in the pediatric population.[6] To address this problem, the authors consider a function-based framework to evaluate SM use, focused on usage patterns as well as related risk and resiliency factors. They hope this framework can guide clinical screening, assessment, and intervention in the future.

A FUNCTION-BASED FRAMEWORK FOR UNDERSTANDING USAGE PATTERNS

Since the 1990s, SM modalities have transformed from static Web sites into dynamic and interactive applications with functions such as image sharing.[11] Much of the evidence examining the link between SM usage and mental health indices focuses on "screen time" as the variable mediating this relationship without accounting for other variables captured in it.[8] Relying solely on-screen time is one dimensional and fails to consider the intricacies of their usage.[12] A function-based framework assessment can identify similar SM behaviors across platforms yet remains generalizable and adaptable enough to survive the rapid evolution of the space.[9]

The framework, summarized in **Fig. 1**, allows clinicians to understand the most salient usage variables utilizing the questions "What? How? and Who?". The result is a personalized usage pattern that enables clinicians to probe for potential risk and resiliency factors specific to that adolescent. In this study, we expand upon each of the variables and explain how a clinician can use this framework in depth.

WHAT? IDENTIFYING FUNCTION-BASED PLATFORM ENGAGEMENT

Identifying which platforms a teenager uses, or how much time they spend on them, is only partially helpful.[13] Identifying SM functions provides clinicians with an anchor point to better understand adolescent online activities. While there are various SM functions, our framework focuses on the following 5: (1) social networking (SN), (2) image sharing, (3) video sharing, (4) livestreaming, and (5) messaging.[14] For more detailed descriptions of these functions refer to Sood and Avari[15] After identifying the platforms, a clinician can explore the functions used and content the adolescent enjoys browsing, as illustrated in **Table 1**. To facilitate engagement, a clinician can and should use their computers to look up and co-watch content during the visit.

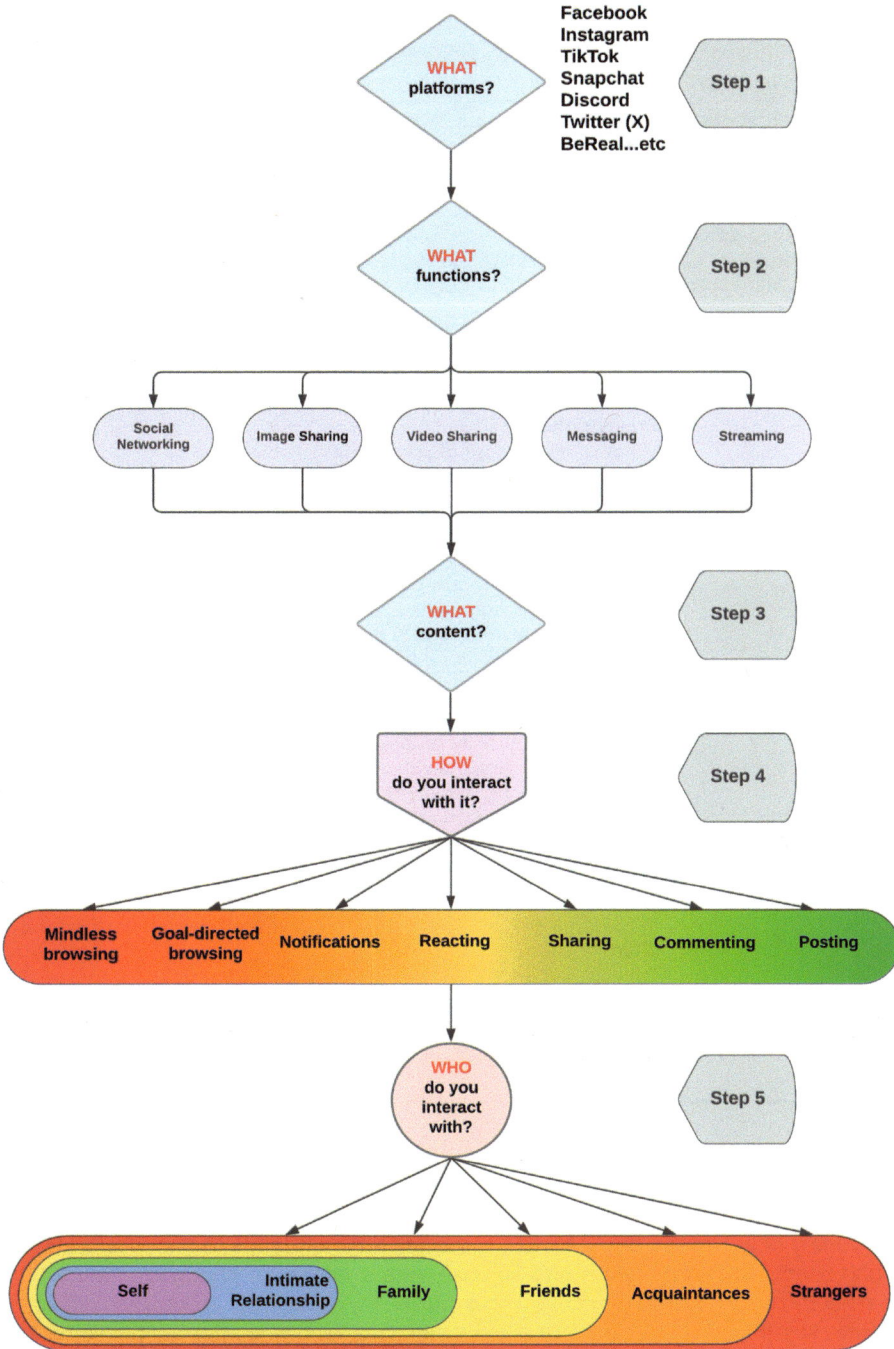

Fig. 1. Social media assessment algorithm.

Table 1
How to identify functions, platforms used, and type of content explored

Step 1: Identify platforms:
- What applications do you use? What is your favorite?
- What app do you spend most time on? How long? What do you mostly do on it?
- What is the latest platform you/your friends have been on? Can you show me how you use it?

Step 2: Identify functions:
- What do you do on SM?
- What features or functions do you like to use the most?
- What are some special features or app functions that you enjoy? Can you show me how they are used?

Step 3: Explore topics of interest within each function:

Social Networking	• What are some of the stories that show up on your feed? • What does your profile page look like? Can you share it with me on your phone? • What is the purpose of your profile? • Do you use [platform] to form friendships? Learn about opportunities? For education?
Image Sharing	• What kind of profiles do you follow? • Is there specific content that you are interested in? • What is the most recent picture you shared? • Do you like viewing pictures of people? Animals? Memes? • What is your favorite photo that you shared, posted, or discovered? • Any specific filters you use?
Video Sharing	• What comes up on your feed? Can you show me some of your favorite videos? • Do you prefer shorter or longer videos? • What are your favorite video topics? • Do you follow any activity-specific accounts? • Do you watch to learn about concepts, events, or ideas? • What other information do you get from videos? • What topics do you post about?
Live Streaming	• What streaming topics do you enjoy watching? • What streaming activities do you find yourself getting notifications from? • Do you ever go live? What do you talk about or do?
Messaging	• What do you message about? • Do you have a special topic that you follow on SM? • Are there things you talk about on SM that you do not talk about in person?

HOW? THE SPECTRUM OF ENGAGEMENT: EXAMINING SOCIAL MEDIA USAGE BEHAVIOR FROM SCROLLING TO POSTING

The variety of activities offered by SM platforms naturally leads to the stratification of young users based on their "types of use" onto a spectrum of engagement.[16] This continuum can be conceptualized in the bidirectional concept of consumption and contribution (**Fig. 2**). *Consumption* is the process of receiving information via various forms of media such as video or images. This is analogous to passive SM use.[17] *Contribution* consists of active SM use such as engagement with and creation of content, including "liking," commenting, sharing, posting, and "going live."[18]

Most adolescents engage in both consumption and contribution behaviors. Consumptive SM use can take form in 2 ways: mindless scrolling and goal-directed

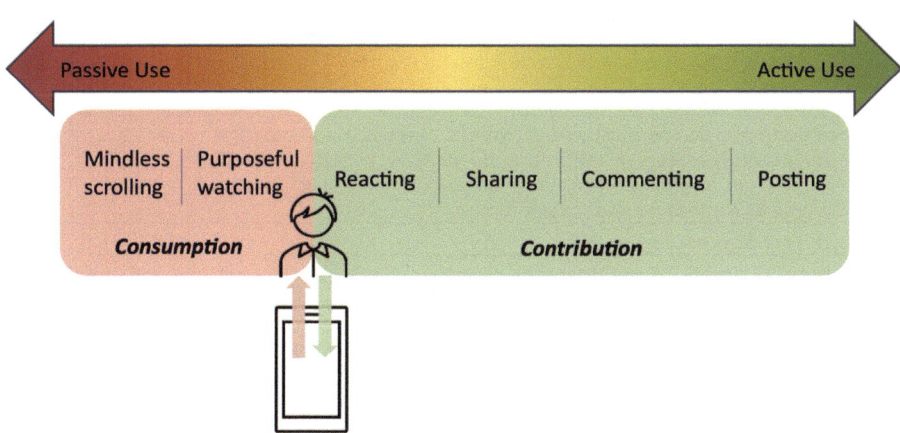

Fig. 2. Spectrum of engagement, evaluating how adolescents interact with social media functions.

browsing. Scrolling through a personalized homepage without purpose has been associated with negative emotions.[19,20] On the other hand, seeking out meaningful connections or content may be related to positive emotions and development.[21] When evaluating contribution, a clinician should differentiate the extent and frequency of engagement. Reacting to and sharing videos provide a different level of social exposure than posting original content and therefore have different risk profiles.[16] Examining ways in which adolescents interact on SM will assist a clinician in identifying risk and resilience factors associated with each type of use.[22] **Table 2** offers questions that will assist in characterizing these patterns of usage.

WHO? ASSESSING RELATIONAL INTERACTIONS ON SOCIAL MEDIA

Adolescents engage in a wide range of online exchanges, ranging from intimate interactions to cursory engagements with online strangers. During these exchanges, they are actively exposed to content shaped not only by their interests, but also by the individuals they follow.[23] As a clinician, characterizing these online interactions can shed light on how adolescents perceive themselves.

Differentiating between the types of interactions, that is, public (acquaintances, strangers) versus private (friends, family), is helpful in further stratifying risk and resilience factors associated with an adolescent's SM use.[23,24] Lyyra and colleagues[23] analyzed data collected from Finnish adolescents as part of the Health Behavior in School-aged Children study in 2018 and found that 22% of adolescents communicated with friends they met through the Internet and 13% reported online communication with complete strangers. In that same study, the authors discovered that online communication with people adolescents know in person was correlated with positive outcomes while communication with online friends or strangers was negatively associated with well-being indicators measured such as loneliness, and problematic SM use. Conversely, some authors argue that, particularly in marginalized populations such as lesbian, gay, bisexual, transgender and queer (LGBTQ) adolescents, interacting with strangers in supportive communities provides a safe space to learn more about themselves, form friendships, and gain information about sexual health.[25] Further research is required to evaluate the complex relationship between these interactions and mental health indices. **Table 3** offers questions that aid in exploring these relationships.

Table 2
Identify how an adolescent utilizes a function

General questions:

- When using SM, do you mostly view content, react to it, or post it?
- Do you view other people's content, or do you post your own material?
- Do you react or comment on content? Do you share content?
- What type of content do you engage with?

Function-specific questions

Social Networking	• Do you spend time looking at other people's profiles and updates? • Have you posted any content on your timeline or anyone else's? • How often do you check your [platform] newsfeed? • How often do you engage with your followers? How do you do that? • Do you feel like your profile is an accurate representation of yourself? • Do you mostly look at other people's profiles and updates or do you react and post?
Image Sharing	• How often do you look at images on [platform]? How often do you react to them? • How often do you comment on pictures? • Do you post your own pictures and/or share other people's image content? • Do you post pictures of yourself? Family? Friends? Hobbies or interests? • Do you uncontrollably scroll through images? • Do you edit or use filters for your pictures? • Do other people react to your pictures? Share it? Comment on it? How does that make you feel?
Video Sharing	• Do you create content? Could you share with me some of your videos? • Do you watch videos or do you also react (like or heart) to videos? • Do you comment on a video? How often? • Do you share videos with other people? • What type of content do you create? • Do you watch videos with a goal in mind?
Live Streaming	• Do you mostly lurk or do you interact with streamers? • Are you someone who streams? How often? How long? • What content do you post? • Do you get paid for your streaming? • Have you tipped a streamer? • How often do you watch? How long?
Direct Messaging	• Do you post messages or send texts? • Do you read blogs or messages by others? • Do you share messages or text produced by others (like retweeting)? • How often do you message others? How much time do you spend texting? • Do you text others first? Or do people message you first?
Special Features	• Help me understand how [function] works. • What is your longest streak on [platform: BeReal or Snapchat]? • Is there a special feature specific to [insert platform]? How do you use it?

WHY? A NUANCED ASSESSMENT OF PROTECTIVE AND RISK FACTORS BASED ON SOCIAL MEDIA USAGE PROFILE

Integrating knowledge about adolescent SM activity and interaction patterns, a clinician can generally stratify types of use into 4 categories illustrated in **Table 4**: (1) private passive, (2) public passive, (3) private active, and (4) public active. Based

Table 3
Questions to evaluate who the adolescent is interacting with

	Passive Use	Active Use
Social Networking	• Are you a part of specific groups? Do you feel like you belong? • Do you follow certain accounts? Can you show me their content? • Do you check in or read updates from anyone more frequently than others?	• Who do you mostly interact with on SM? • Are you an influencer? Do you have a lot of followers? • Do you have different accounts? • Do you ever interact with anyone you have not met in person?
Image Sharing	• Who do you receive images from? • Who do you mostly follow? • Who makes up the people you follow? Friends? Strangers? • Do you receive images from people you do not know?	• Who do you mostly send pictures to? • Do you ever send images to people you do not know? • Are your images private or public? • Do you have different accounts you share pictures on? • Do you have fake profiles? Share images anonymously?
Video Sharing	• Whose videos do you mostly watch? • Do you privately receive videos from others? If so, from who? • How do you discover new video content? • Who mostly shows up on your homepage? Friends? Influencers? Strangers? • Do you have creators or communities that you follow?	• Who do you share your own videos with? • Do you collaborate with users to create videos? • Do you ever tag other people in videos you create? Do you ever get tagged? • How often do you post public videos vs private videos? • Do you post content for communities?
Live Streaming	• Which streamers do you follow? Friends, online strangers? • How do you find new streamers? • Who are your favorite streamers? Do you know them personally? • Do you belong to any communities?	• Who do you mostly interact with during live content? • Do you ever join live streams? If so, with who? • Do you have an audience or followers? Who typically watches you? • Do you ever donate money to live streamers?
Messaging	• Are you part of any messaging groups or communities? • Who do you most frequently message? • Have you ever received messages from people you do not know? • Do you know the people you are interacting with via text? • Do you prefer individual chats or group chats? • When in group chats, do you engage and participate in the conversations?	

on empirical data and anecdotal reports, each type of use is associated with certain risk and resilience factors. This section delves into some of these factors shown in **Table 5**, how they may present across functions of SM, and how they may be elicited.[12,21,26]

Social Networking

SN enables adolescents to interact with individuals within and outside of their traditionally defined social circles.[27] Through such connections, adolescents foster deep connections and combat isolation.[5] However, online interactions may come at the expense of offline relationships, often hindering development of social skills and contributing to loneliness.[28] While establishing online connections with family and friends can help adolescents maintain strong relationships, constant connection can fuel fear of missing out (colloquially: FOMO), leading to feelings of inadequacy and dissatisfaction.[29]

In addition to fostering a sense of connection, SN can provide adolescents with a platform to explore and express their identity and share thoughts, feelings, and experiences in supportive spaces.[12,26] This can empower adolescents, especially underrepresented minorities, and contribute to their positive self-development.[30,31] However, the public nature of these activities can increase the risk of shaming, harassment, and cyberbullying, all which are associated with negative mental health outcomes and internalizing symptoms of depression and anxiety.[32,33]

Finally, through SN, adolescents encounter opinions, experiences, and narratives beyond that of their immediate social circles. While this may broaden their worldview and foster curiosity in certain instances, it could also lead to the creation of echo chambers, where one directional adolescent beliefs are reinforced.[34]

Image Sharing

Image sharing provides adolescents with a canvas for self-expression. Whether posting snapshots of their daily lives, or sharing funny memes, adolescents rely on image-sharing function to develop their identities and nurture creativity. Through exploring connections outside of their social circles, adolescents can seek inspiration and learn about art, culture, and different ways of expression. However, this same process that facilitates creative expression can also result in anxiety, negative self-perception, and fear of judgment as the adolescent's identity is vulnerable to public criticism.[35] Adolescents viewing flawless portrayals and embellishments of others also increase upward social comparison and body image concerns, decreasing mental well-being and possibly leading to eating disorder behaviors.[36]

More privately, image sharing among close peers can be used as a mean of communication.[37] However, as illustrated earlier, sharing pictures is a double-edged sword, even when done among peers. While this more emotive approach of communication can provide a sense of intimacy and connection, it can also be used to share inappropriate content including nudity, often without consent.[38–40]

Video Sharing

Much like image sharing, video sharing promotes both creative expression and consumption of video content. Video creation offers youth an outlet where they can share their identities fully compared to snapshots via image sharing. However, time involved in video creation compared to image creation is often longer due to preparation, production, and editing of video content. As a result, young creators can develop lower self-esteem in response to their public videos receiving less views compared to others, a phenomenon known as upward social comparison,

Table 4
Profile-specific risk and resilience factors categorized by pattern of use and interaction

How Who	Consumption (*Passive Use: Mindless Browsing, Goal-directed Engagement*)	Contribution (*Active Use: Engaging, Reacting, Posting*)
Risk Factors Associated with SM Use Patterns		
Private	Fear of missing out (FOMO)	Drama and conflict
	Comparison trap	Pressure to conform
	Filter bubble	Negative self-presentation
	Passive loneliness	External source of validation
	Conformity pressure	Social exclusion
	Cyberbullying	Nudity/sexting/sexual coercion
Public	FOMO	Reputation damage
	Comparison trap	Cyberbullying/harassment
	Exposure to harmful content	Creation fatigue (burnout)
	Time sink	Oversharing (location, financial
	Scams and catfishing	information)
	Contagion	Privacy violation (blackmail,
	Misinformation	exploiting media content)
	Body image and unrealistic expectations	Unsolicited attention/grooming
	Pornography	Pressure to perform
	Addiction	Body image
	Secondary bullying	Sharing harmful content
Resilience Factors Associated with SM Use Patterns		
Private	Selective connection	Community and connection
	Staying connected	Safe spaces
	Shared experience	Maintaining friendships
	Belonging	Prosocial behavior
	Social and emotional support	Socialization and communication skills
		Networking
Public	Exposure to diverse perspectives	Community and connection
	Inspiration and motivation	Expression and creativity
	Entertainment and discovery	Challenging stereotypes
	Learning from experts/education	Minority spaces
	Illness support	Social connection and validation
	Fact-checking	Activism
	Positive community	Boosting self-confidence

discussed earlier.[41] Ironically, upward social comparison often leads young users to increase watching content that exacerbates their poor self-esteem, creating a vicious cycle.[42]

Video sharing for passive consumers also entails education. Youth often turn to YouTube and TikTok to learn about current events, which allows informed decision-making regarding personal beliefs. This can often translate into informed action such donating to charity and becoming involved with local, national, or international communities. However, increased passive video consumption can alternatively lead to doom scrolling, where users obsessively seek negative and depressing information on SM. Doom scrolling has been shown to have positive correlations with FOMO and SM addiction.[43,44] Dangerous trends, where users try to popularize hazardous behavior to generate viewership, are new fads permeating video-sharing platforms.[45] Trends in the form of online challenges may involve the ingestion of large amounts of substances (Benadryl, cinnamon), which has led to hospitalizations and deaths among adolescents.[46,47]

Direct Messaging

Messaging serves as a direct form of communication among adolescents in SM, particularly during the coronavirus disease 2019 (COVID-19) pandemic.[28,48] Direct messaging can promote a feeling of inclusion, which plays an essential role in adolescent development.[48] However, there are also significant risks to direct messaging. Cyberbullying is prevalent in SM, with 1 in 6 high school students endorsing victimization.[49] Risk factors for victims include endorsement of loneliness and social anxiety while those who perpetrate cyberbullying have often been previous perpetrators of traditional bullying. Direct messaging examples of cyberbullying include verbal violence (insulting or offensive direct messages), group violence (exclusion from group chats or group verbal violence), cyberstalking (harassing individuals continually via direct messaging), and sexual violence (unwanted sexually explicit messages sent to users without their consent).[32,38,40] Victims of cyberbullying are 1.9 times more likely to attempt suicide.[49]

Sexual exploration, a common adolescent phenomenon, has expanded to the digital space. Female individuals receive sexts (sexual texts) at a higher rate than male individuals. While only older youth are more likely to send sexts, both younger and older adolescents receive sexts at similar rates.[50] The ephemeral nature of disappearing direct messages on Snapchat adds to the allure of sending sexually explicit

Table 5
Negative experiences associated with social media use and questions to assess for these factors adopted from Smahel colleagues[56]

Overall negative experiences	• Has anything ever happened online that bothered or upset you in some way (eg, made you feel upset, uncomfortable, scared, or that you should not have seen it)?
Cyberbullying and harassment	• Has anyone even treated you in hurtful or nasty ways (teasing or making fun of you, leaving you out of things)? How often did this happen? Did you know them?
Harmful content	• Sometimes people discuss things that may not be good for you like ways of hurting yourself or ending your life, ways to be thin, racism, drug abuse, violence. Have you seen online content or online discussions where people talk about or show any of these things?
Privacy and data misuse	• Has anybody used your personal information in ways you did not like? Used your password and pretended to be you? Created information about you that was mean or hostile? Found out where you lived by tracking your phone?
Addiction	• Has an online activity become the most important part of your life? Made you feel better? Had to do more of that activity to feel better? Had unpleasant feelings after stopping the activity? Had significant disagreement with parents associated with activity? Or failed to reduce or stop spending time doing the activity?
Sexting	• Sometimes people may send sexual messages or images or videos. By this, we mean talk about having sex or images of people naked or images of people having sex. Have you ever received/sent any similar content? From/to who? How often? Was it unsolicited or unwanted? Has anyone asked you for sexual information about yourself?
Porn and explicit material	• Have you seen images that may show people naked or people having sex or engaging in sexual activities?

Table 6
Excerpt from interview with patient based on the framework

Step of Framework	Interview
What platform?	*Clinician: Hey Caleb, what have you been up to on SM lately? What are your favorite apps?* *Patient:* Mostly Snapchat and TikTok
What function?	*Clinician:* Cool! How do you use Snapchat? I know there are a ton of features on there. *Patient:* I message a lot of my friends on Snapchat. We try to keep our snap streaks going. *Clinician:* Do you use TikTok the same way? *Patient:* Not really. I basically scroll through videos for hours late at night
What content?	*Clinician:* It seems like both Snapchat and TikTok are important to you. What do you typically talk about on Snapchat? Do you send the same messages to everyone? *Patient:* Well, I mostly talk about gossip and stuff at school. There is this guy I have been messaging, which is a bit different than my other friend groups. *Clinician:* And do you and your friends as well as this guy all follow the same videos on TikTok as well? What comes up on your "For You" page? *Patient:* I am not sure what shows up for them, but I am getting really into fashion, and models, or what apparel they are wearing comes up a lot while scrolling.
How do you engage?	*Clinician:* Sounds like you are pretty active in Snapchat but maybe more of a scroller on TikTok? *Patient:* Yeah, I am almost always texting my friends on Snapchat. I do not really create any content or anything, so I more scroll all the time. I am not putting myself out to the public like that. But like I watch so many videos, it is killing my sleep. *Clinician:* You mentioned earlier that you message a lot of people on Snapchat. How big do these groups get? *Patient:* Well, there is a school group which is like 20 people, but I more so just enjoy the drama there and do not contribute. We have a smaller group of 4–5 people that is my core group, and we all have streaks together independently. I did leave the group for a little bit because it got a bit toxic. People were saying some really annoying stuff. Then I have a private chat with this guy my friends introduced me to on the app. He is super nice but lives out of state.
Who do you interact with?	*Clinician:* So it sounds like on Snapchat you have your primary group of friends and maybe a romantic interest? *Patient:* Haha, you can say that. On Snapchat, my friends Rose, Jayden, and Daniel are the ones who I interact with the most. I have known them since middle school. The guy whom I like is named Josh. He likes fashion like me, and he is hilarious. *Clinician:* And on TikTok, you mostly scroll, but do you ever comment on anyone's videos? *Patient:* Oh, absolutely not. I enjoy the content, but I do not want to be in the public eye whatsoever. Maybe 1 day, I could post some of my designs but that is far off.
Risk and resilience factors?	*Clinician:* I have really enjoyed getting to know you! It really seems like you have deep meaningful connections with your friends on Snapchat and your passion for fashion is developing through TikTok. Very cool!

(continued on next page)

Table 6 *(continued)*	
Step of Framework	**Interview**
	Patient: Thanks!
	Clinician: As your doctor, one of my jobs is to highlight aspects of safety as well when it comes to SM use. I noticed that Josh, on Snapchat, is important to you. I also notice that he is someone you may not have met and you are romantically interested in him. Have you both engaged in sexting at all?
	Patient: Yeah, sometimes.
	Clinician: Thanks for letting me know. Do you ever feel pressured to send sexts?
	Patient: Not really. We just started that and he does not pressure me. But my friends are always talking about it, and what they do, and I feel like I am falling behind.
	Clinician: It is totally normal to feel like you have to keep up with everyone, especially when it comes to more intimate stuff. Are you open to having a conversation on how we can keep you safe?

messages and photos via direct messaging. Under the guise of disappearing messages, adolescents may be subject to sexual coercion in the form of unwanted requests for sexually explicit images.[38,40] By 15, 1 in 5 teens experience sexual coercion via direct messaging.[51]

Streaming

Live streaming serves as a powerful tool that encourages adolescent self-expression in the same way image and video sharing does, allowing adolescents to showcase their talents and skills while connecting real time with their audience.[52] As a result, adolescents who engage in these activities find themselves contributing to supportive communities and fostering a sense of belonging across viewers. On the other hand, the pressure to perform and maintain engagement can be overwhelming for adolescents, contributing to burnout, anxiety, and other negative mental health indices.[53] Additionally, due to its public and real-time nature, adolescent streamers may be exposed to criticism, harassment, and cyberbullying in much more direct manner.

Viewing live streams can be gratifying and entertaining for many adolescents who are part of specific communities or follow certain influencers. Highly curated streams provide educational content and positive role modeling, which leads to improve well-being and communication skills.[54] However, with limited moderation, adolescents may end up being exposed to harmful content, such as violence and hate speech.[55]

To assess for negative experiences and risks associated with SM across functions, a clinician can refer to **Table 5** for possible questions to ask based on EU Kids Online 2020 report by Smahel and colleagues.[56]

FROM THEORY TO PRACTICE: PUTTING THE FRAMEWORK TO ACTION

With this framework in mind, let us revisit our patient, Caleb, and illustrate an example of how to formulate an assessment of his SM use, highlighting potential risky behaviors as well as protective factors in his interactions. The interview is categorized based on the previously delineated framework and described in **Table 6**.

Caleb's SM use leans more toward the consumption side of the engagement spectrum with video sharing on TikTok, while active engagement occurs within his immediate social circles on Snapchat. Consulting **Table 5** reveals several potential risk and resilience factors associated with Caleb's pattern of SM use. Protective factors include finding inspiration from the content creators he follows on TikTok and support from his friends on Snapchat. Risk factors stemming from private contribution include sexting, which can include sexual coercion and can put youth in harm's way if they are not careful. Additionally, Caleb's excessive public consumption via watching content on TikTok for countless hours is getting in the way of his sleep or other offline activities. There are many other directions that the interview can go, such as body image concerns via the videos Caleb watches or screening for cyberbullying in the setting of his "toxic" interactions. These insights can inform the clinician's follow-up questions, which aim to uncover any harmful experiences Caleb may have encountered or might be at risk of in the future.

SUMMARY

Due to SM's exponential growth, clinicians may feel lost in their assessments of how SM applications may be affecting their patients' well-being. Our framework establishes a time-tested methodology, focusing on the functions of applications rather than applications in a vacuum. Establishing an alliance through assessing which applications are important and what functions are utilized on applications allows clinicians to get a better sense of youth's SM habits. Detailing how youth interact with SM (passive vs active) and who they interact with (private vs public) informs clinicians about youth engagement in SM. Combining habits with engagement leads to stratification of protective and risk factors. These factors will then dictate how clinicians can guide youth in reducing dangerous SM habits while reinforcing positive influences.

By no means is this framework exhaustive nor does it evaluate every facet of adolescent SM behavior. What we have learned over the decade is that SM behavior is much more complex than initially thought. Furthermore, technology advances much faster than peer-reviewed clinical research data, forcing clinicians to stay up-to-date with youth technological use. We hope that this guide serves as a scaffolding that can be adapted in later years when new SM giants have taken hold.

CLINICS CARE POINTS

Elicit Specific Social Media Use Patterns:
- Instead of only asking about screen time, clinicians should assess the specific functions of social media use (eg, messaging, video sharing) to identify personalized risk and resilience factors.

Passive vs. Active Use:
- Differentiate between passive consumption (e.g., scrolling) and active participation (eg, posting). Passive use can be linked with negative emotions, while active use may offer social connection but also risks like cyberbullying.

Identify Relational Interactions:
- Explore who adolescents interact with online—whether with known peers or strangers. Public interactions, particularly with strangers, can pose greater risks, such as exposure to harmful content or privacy violations.

Assess for Hidden Risks:
- Look for signs of risky behaviors, such as sexting, cyberbullying, or exposure to harmful content. These interactions can occur privately and may not be immediately visible without targeted questioning.

Evaluate Impact on Offline Life:
- Excessive social media use, especially during late hours, can negatively impact sleep and offline activities. Clinicians should assess how social media is affecting the patient's daily functioning.

Screen for Vulnerabilities in High-Risk Groups:
- Pay attention to marginalized or vulnerable adolescents, such as LGBTQ youth, who may find community support online but are also at risk of harassment or cyberbullying.

Promote Safe Use and Resilience:
- Highlight protective factors, like creative expression and supportive online communities, while providing guidance on reducing exposure to harmful content and risky behaviors.

DISCLOSURE

The authors have no conflicts to disclose.

REFERENCES

1. Teens, social media and technology 2023. Pew Research Center: Internet, Science & Tech; 2023. Available at: https://www.pewresearch.org/internet/2023/12/11/teens-social-media-and-technology-2023/. Accessed December 20, 2023.
2. The common sense Census: media use by tweens and teens. Common Sense Media; 2021. Available at: https://www.commonsensemedia.org/research/the-common-sense-census-media-use-by-tweens-and-teens-2021. Accessed February 9, 2024.
3. Teens spend average of 4.8 hours on social media per day. Available at: https://news.gallup.com/poll/512576/teens-spend-average-hours-social-media-per-day.aspx. Accessed February 9, 2024.
4. The need to belong: desire for interpersonal attachments as a fundamental human motivation. Available at: https://psycnet.apa.org/record/1995-29052-001. Accessed February 9, 2024.
5. Orben A, Tomova L, Blakemore SJ. The effects of social deprivation on adolescent development and mental health. Lancet Child Adolesc Health 2020;4(8):634–40.
6. Odgers CL, Jensen MR. Annual research review: adolescent mental health in the digital age: facts, fears, and future directions. J Child Psychol Psychiatry 2020;61(3):336–48.
7. Orben A, Przybylski AK, Blakemore SJ, et al. Windows of developmental sensitivity to social media. Nat Commun 2022;13:1649.
8. Valkenburg PM, Meier A, Beyens I. Social media use and its impact on adolescent mental health: an umbrella review of the evidence. Curr Opin Psychol 2022;44:58–68.
9. Trifiro BM, Gerson J. Social media usage patterns: research note regarding the lack of universal validated measures for active and passive use. Soc Media Soc 2019;5(2):2056305119848743.
10. Ortiz-Ospina E, Roser M. The rise of social media. Our World in Data 2023. Available at: https://ourworldindata.org/rise-of-social-media.
11. Mutabazi. The evolution of social media: how did it begin, and where could it go next? | maryville online. Available at: https://online.maryville.edu/blog/evolution-social-media/. Accessed February 9, 2024.
12. Granic I, Morita H, Scholten H. Beyond screen time: identity development in the digital age. Psychol Inq 2020;31(3):195–223.

13. Odgers CL, Jensen MR. Adolescent development and growing divides in the digital age. Dialogues Clin Neurosci 2020;22(2):143–9.

14. Quesenberry K. Social media update: top social media channels by category. 2021. Available at: https://www.postcontrolmarketing.com/social-media-update-top-social-media-channels-by-category/.

15. Sood A, Avari JM. Social media and screen time in the clinical interview: what to ask and what it means?. In: Spaniardi A, Avari JM, editors. Teens, screens, and social connection. Cham: Springer; 2023. https://doi.org/10.1007/978-3-031-24804-7_2.

16. Beyens I, Pouwels JL, Van Driel II, et al. Social media use and adolescents' well-being: developing a typology of person-specific effect patterns. Commun Res 2021. https://doi.org/10.1177/00936502211038196.

17. Examining the effects of passive WeChat use in China: international journal of human–computer interaction: vol 35, No 17. Available at: https://www.tandfonline.com/doi/abs/10.1080/10447318.2018.1559535. Accessed February 9, 2024.

18. Gerson J, Plagnol AC, Corr PJ. Passive and active Facebook use measure (PAUM): validation and relationship to the reinforcement sensitivity theory. Pers Indiv Differ 2017;117:81–90.

19. Ding Q, Zhang YX, Wei H, et al. Passive social network site use and subjective well-being among Chinese university students: a moderated mediation model of envy and gender. Pers Indiv Differ 2017;113:142–6.

20. Sinha S, Sharma MK, Tadpatrikar A, et al. Scrolling Mindlessly: emerging mental health implications of social networking sites. Journal of Public Health and Primary Care 2023;4(3):179–81.

21. Naslund JA, Bondre A, Torous J, et al. Social media and mental health: benefits, risks, and opportunities for research and practice. J Technol Behav Sci 2020;5(3):245–57.

22. Scarpulla E, Stosic MD, Weaver AE, et al. Should I post? The relationships among social media use, emotion recognition, and mental health. Front Psychol 2023;14:1161300.

23. Lyyra N, Junttila N, Gustafsson J, et al. Adolescents' online communication and well-being: findings from the 2018 health behavior in school-aged children (HBSC) study. Front Psychiatry 2022;13:976404. Available at: https://www.frontiersin.org/journals/psychiatry/articles/10.3389/fpsyt.2022.976404.

24. Nesi J, Telzer EH, Prinstein MJ. Adolescent development in the digital media context. Psychol Inq 2020;31(3):229–34.

25. Berger MN, Taba M, Marino JL, et al. Social media's role in support networks among LGBTQ adolescents: a qualitative study. Sex Health 2021;18(5):421–31.

26. Popat A, Tarrant C. Exploring adolescents' perspectives on social media and mental health and well-being – a qualitative literature review. Clin Child Psychol Psychiatry 2023;28(1):323–37.

27. Pew Research Center. Internet, science & tech. Chapter 4: social media and friendships. 2015. Available at: https://www.pewresearch.org/internet/2015/08/06/chapter-4-social-media-and-friendships/.

28. Charmaraman L, Lynch AD, Richer AM, et al. Examining early adolescent positive and negative social technology behaviors and well-being during the COVID-19 pandemic. Technol Mind Behav 2022;3(1). https://doi.org/10.1037/tmb0000062.

29. Martino J, Pegg J, Frates EP. The connection prescription: using the power of social interactions and the deep desire for connectedness to empower health and wellness. Am J Lifestyle Med 2015;11(6):466–75.

30. Brough M, Literat I, Ikin A. 'Good social media?': underrepresented youth perspectives on the ethical and equitable design of social media platforms. Soc Media Soc 2020;6(2):2056305120928488.

31. How social media platforms can empower disabled women – women's eNews. Available at: https://womensenews.org/2024/02/how-social-media-platforms-can-empower-disabled-women/. Accessed February 9, 2024.

32. Schade BP, Larwin KH, Larwin DA. Public vs. private cyberbullying among adolescents. Interdiscip Educ Psychol 2017;1(1). https://doi.org/10.31532/Interdiscip EducPsychol.1.1.005.

33. Khalaf AM, Alubied AA, Khalaf AM, et al. The impact of social media on the mental health of adolescents and young adults: a systematic review. Cureus 2023;15(8). https://doi.org/10.7759/cureus.42990.

34. Cinelli M, De Francisci Morales G, Galeazzi A, et al. The echo chamber effect on social media. Proc Natl Acad Sci U S A 2021;118(9). https://doi.org/10.1073/pnas.2023301118.

35. Jiang S, Ngien A. The effects of Instagram use, social comparison, and self-esteem on social anxiety: a survey study in Singapore. Soc Media Soc 2020; 6(2). https://doi.org/10.1177/2056305120912488.

36. Tiggemann M, Anderberg I. Social media is not real: the effect of 'Instagram vs reality' images on women's social comparison and body image. New Media Soc 2020;22(12):2183–99.

37. Russmann U, Svensson J. Introduction to visual communication in the age of social media: conceptual, theoretical and methodological challenges. Media Commun 2017;5(4):1–5.

38. Mori C, Park J, Temple JR, et al. Are youth sexting rates still on the rise? A meta-analytic update. J Adolesc Health 2022;70(4):531–9.

39. Fung IC, Blankenship EB, Ahweyevu JO, et al. Public health implications of image-based social media: a systematic review of Instagram, pinterest, tumblr, and flickr. Perm J 2020;24(18):307.

40. Thulin EJ, Kernsmith P, Fleming PJ, et al. Coercive-sexting: predicting adolescent initial exposure to electronic coercive sexual dating violence. Comput Human Behav 2023;141:107641.

41. Verduyn P, Gugushvili N, Massar K, et al. Social comparison on social networking sites. Curr Opin Psychol 2020;36:32–7.

42. Vogel EA, Rose JP, Roberts LR, et al. Social comparison, social media, and self-esteem. Psychol Pop Media Cult 2014;3(4):206–22.

43. McLaughlin B, Gotlieb M, Mills D. Caught in a dangerous world: problematic news consumption and its relationship to mental and physical ill-being. Health Commun 2022;38(12):1590–601.

44. Satici SA, Tekin EG, Deniz ME, et al. Doomscrolling scale: its association with personality traits, psychological distress, social media use, and wellbeing. Appl Res Qual Life 2023;18(2):833–47.

45. Bonifazi G, Cecchini S, Corradini E, et al. Investigating community evolutions in TikTok dangerous and non-dangerous challenges. J Inf Sci 2022. 016555152211165.

46. Atherton RR. The 'nutmeg challenge': a dangerous social media trend. Arch Dis Child 2021;106(5):517–8.

47. Kriegel ER, Lazarevic B, Athanasian CE, et al. TikTok, tide pods and tiger king: health implications of trends taking over pediatric populations. Curr Opin Pediatr 2021;33(1):170–7.

48. Ehrenreich SE, Meter DJ, Beron KJ, et al. How adolescents use text messaging through their high school years. J Res Adolesc 2020;30(2):521–40.

49. Alavi N, Reshetukha T, Prost E, et al. Relationship between bullying and suicidal behaviour in youth presenting to the emergency department. J Can Acad Child Adolesc Psychiatry 2017;26(2):70–7.
50. Choi H, Van Ouytsel J, Temple JR. Association between sexting and sexual coercion among female adolescents. J Adolesc 2016;53:164–8.
51. Morrison-Beedy D, Grove L. Adolescent girls' experiences with sexual pressure, coercion, and victimization: #MeToo. Worldviews Evid Based Nurs 2018;15(3): 225–9.
52. A short guide to live streaming. Available at: https://www.thinkuknow.co.uk/parents/articles/what-is-live-streaming/. Accessed February 10, 2024.
53. Woodcock J, Johnson MR. The affective labor and performance of live streaming on twitch. Tv. Television & New Media 2019;20(8):813–23.
54. Wit JD, van der Kraan A, Theeuwes J. Live streams on twitch help viewers cope with difficult periods in life. Front Psychol 2020;11:586975.
55. Cabeza-Ramírez LJ, Fuentes-García FJ, Muñoz-Fernandez GA. Exploring the emerging domain of research on video game live streaming in web of science: state of the art, changes and trends. Int J Environ Res Public Health 2021; 18(6):2917.
56. Smahel D, Machackova H, Mascheroni G, et al. EU Kids online 2020: survey results from 19 countries. EU Kids Online 2020. https://doi.org/10.21953/lse.47fdeqj01ofo.

Paging Dr Influencer
Social Media & Psychiatric Self-Diagnosis

Bushra Rizwan, MD[a,b,*], Paul E. Weigle, MD[c]

KEYWORDS

- Social media • Self-diagnosis • Adolescents

KEY POINTS

- Youth frequently use social media to learn about mental health and understand their own experiences.
- Mental health misinformation on social media posts is common, as entertainment is prioritized over accuracy or authoritative sources.
- The process of self-diagnosis in adolescents is complex and often misguided, and can help meet psychological needs in an unhealthy fashion.
- Clinicians evaluating youth who self-diagnose should understand the source and function of these beliefs, and verify symptoms via collateral sources.

OVERVIEW AND BACKGROUND

Self-diagnosis is the process of identifying health conditions in oneself.[1] Individuals compare information learned about psychiatric or medical conditions from digital resources, books, and testimonials of others to their own experiences to self-diagnose. This process can be beneficial, but misdiagnosis is common, and fraught with a myriad of potential problems including over-identification with the illness, contagion, or pursuing inappropriate and possibly harmful treatments.

In this review, we discuss clinical experience and research evidence concerning the phenomenon of adolescent self-diagnosis via social media. Adolescents increasingly go online to learn about mental health and understand their own experiences.[2] One the one hand, social media facilitates open, semi-public discussions about mental illness which can spread awareness and reduce stigma. Mental health posts can

[a] Division of Child and Adolescent Psychiatry, Department of Psychiatry and Behavioral Sciences, Johns Hopkins Hospital, 1800 Orleans Street, Baltimore, MD 21287, USA; [b] Department of Developmental Behavioral Health, Kennedy Krieger Institute, 1741 Ashland Avenue, Baltimore, MD 21205, USA; [c] Department of Psychiatry, University of Connecticut School of Medicine, 352 Mansfield Road, Storrs, CT 06269, USA
* Corresponding author. Division of Child and Adolescent Psychiatry, Department of Psychiatry and Behavioral Sciences, Johns Hopkins Hospital, Baltimore.
E-mail address: brizwan1@jhmi.edu

Pediatr Clin N Am 72 (2025) 267–278
https://doi.org/10.1016/j.pcl.2024.09.003　　　　　　**pediatric.theclinics.com**
0031-3955/25/© 2024 Elsevier Inc. All rights reserved, including those for text and data mining, AI training, and similar technologies.

facilitate access to valuable mental health information and resources, but related negative consequences must be considered. The growth of social media has created a platform for mass and targeted psychoeducation which is often sensationalized, misleading, or false. Claims about mental illness made on social media posts often contain misinformation,[3] as platforms do not verify content and often fail to censor harmful posts, which perpetuates misinformation and encourages unproven treatments. Misinformation can lead vulnerable youth to incorrectly identify with specific psychiatric illness, pursue inappropriate treatments or delay seeking evidence-based treatments, and result in significant harm.

SOCIAL MEDIA & CHILD AND ADOLESCENT PSYCHIATRY

Social media can be easily accessed through smart phones and other personal electronic devices and allows for immediate connection. Research studies have shown that 96% of youth are constantly connected to the internet.[4] Adolescents have been avid adopters of social media; most have quickly incorporated it as a fundamental part of their daily lives. One recent survey of over 1500 US adolescents found they averaged 4.8 hours per day on social media.[5] Children and adolescents may be most susceptible to social media content due to key aspects of psychosocial development and social learning.

Social interactions are an integral part of the human experience and our success as a species. Early humans used cave paintings, petroglyphs, and hieroglyphs to communicate information and ideas, predecessors to the modern-day use of social media platforms and emojis.[6] Social interactions allow for the division of labor and scaffolding learned experiences to create culture and pass on knowledge vital for survival. A substantial portion of our brain is devoted to language and social processing for precisely these reasons. At no point in the human lifespan is socialization more important than in childhood and adolescence. Social learning theory posits that youth learn how to behave through observation, imitation, and modeling, a process historically done in person, but increasingly through screen media.[7] The adolescent mind is especially oriented toward the behavior and reactions of one's peers. Social media is an increasingly important medium for social learning as teens spend as much time on social media observing interactions of peers as they do in-person. People are more likely to imitate behaviors and ideas of those of higher social status, a concept known as prestige bias.

It is important to review Erik Erikson's model of psychosocial development to provide a conceptual framework for understanding specific vulnerability in youth. In late childhood (age 7–12), children typically develop a sense of industry, reinforcing confidence in their abilities to accomplish tasks and contribute to peer groups. Children compare their abilities and achievements to same age peers, which helps build their sense of industry. Meanwhile, adolescent years (age 12–18) are focused on identity formation. Peer influence, acceptance, and belonging are key psychosocial developmental milestones for adolescents.[8] Prior to the advent of social media, children and adolescents developed these skills in in-person unstructured play and socializing as well as in school and through organized sports and extracurricular activities. The ability to connect with peers through social media and related applications ("apps") has altered the arena in which these skills are developed. The psychosocial tasks during this phase of development focus on industry, identity, and role formation.[9] Recent functional MRI studies have revealed significant developmental differences in brain regions associated with social cognition tasks of the adolescent brain compared to that of adults,[10] providing support for Erik Erikson's models.

SOCIAL CONTAGION

The American Association of Psychology defines social contagion as "the spread of behaviors, attitudes, and affect through crowds and other types of social aggregates from one member to another".[11] It builds off observations that were made in ancient times by authors such as Plato, that behaviors can be spread from one person to another through imitation. Also known as sociogenic epidemics, epidemic hysteria, mass hysteria, or culture-bound stress reaction, they consist of a constellation of symptoms that spread between people who share beliefs related to those symptoms, for which anxiety-related symptoms have become typical in modern times.[12] Traditionally spread by face-to-face communication, social contagion is more commonly spread via mass media, increasingly by social media. A wave of popular TikTok posts concerning Tourette's disorder (totaling 6 billion views in 2021) were implicated in an unprecedented concurrent rise of adolescents presenting for treatment of new-onset functional tics, in an apparent case of mass social media contagion.[13] The potential of social media as a vector for social contagion of risky behaviors appears considerable, reviewed in detail by Harness and colleagues (2022) in this issue.[14]

Psychiatric contagion can be partially explained via emotion contagion, the social spread of feelings, and related behaviors. The potential for social media to transmit emotional contagion was demonstrated in an experiment in which the Facebook feed of participants was altered to vary the frequency of stories with a positive or negative emotional tone.[15] Participants exposed to fewer positive expressions produced fewer positive posts and more negative posts themselves. Those exposed to fewer negative expressions posted fewer negative expressions and more positive ones. Although this study showed that social media is capable of transmitting emotions in the short-term, longitudinal research indicates that longer-lasting moods (eg, depression) can be transferred in a similar manner, the strongest effect in females.[16]

The phenomenon of social media contagion is very difficult to study, which accounts for the general lack of scientific evidence about its epidemiology including prevalence. Limited research as suggests the existence of social media transmission of tic-like movements,[17] eating disordered behavior, self-harm,[18] suicidality,[19] dissociative identity disorder,[20] and controversially, gender dysphoria.[21] Evidence provided by all the studies is weak, but it corresponds with the experiences of providers who work with adolescents. At the 2022 Annual Meeting of the American Academy of Child & Adolescent Psychiatry, author Weigle asked attendees "How often do you see patients who seem to believe they suffer from a psychiatric or neurologic condition because of something they saw online?" Of over 100 responders, 74% endorsed "somewhat often" or" very often." Asked "How often do you see teens who seem to be influenced by social media in regards to their sexual and/or gender identity?", 83% responded "somewhat often" or "very often." Our colleagues believe that our patients' symptoms are often a direct reflection of their individual online experiences (eg, social media).

PSYCHIATRIC CONTAGION AND CONVERSION DISORDER VERSUS MALINGERING VERSUS FACTITIOUS DISORDER

Functional neurologic disorder (previously known as conversion disorder), factitious disorder, and malingering are psychiatric diagnoses that differ in involvement of consciousness and motivation. Factitious disorder, categorized under somatic symptoms and related disorders in the Diagnostic and Statistical Manual of Mental Disorders Fifth Edition (DSM-V), involves consciously feigning symptoms to garner medical attention or assume a sick role. Malingering involves intentionally falsifying symptoms for secondary gain, such as financial incentive, or escape from responsibility (ie, to avoid school, work, jail time). Functional neurologic disorder (ie, conversion disorder) differs from malingering and factitious disorder, due to the unconscious origin of the psychological stressor contributing to symptoms and lack of clear motive. The diagnosis of each of these conditions requires that symptoms are not explained by a known neurologic illness, and that clinical findings show clear incompatibility with neurologic symptoms reported by the patient.[22] There is some conceptual overlap between functional neurologic disorders and psychiatric contagion.

Psychiatric contagion, the spread of psychiatric symptoms within a group, can be facilitated by social media platforms where individuals share personal experiences and narratives.[23] Exposure to posts depicting certain symptoms or behaviors may inadvertently influence vulnerable individuals, to mimic or replicate these symptoms themselves for various reasons, demonstrating the complexity of social media and mental health interplay. It is important to understand various motivations for the replication of symptoms, as youth can present with primary, secondary, or unclear motives for self-diagnosis.

Adolescence is a period of identity exploration. Adolescents are often uncertain about their identity and seeking a sense of belonging. Assuming a sick role can provide a stable identity for those who perceive illness as a defining characteristic of self. Those who consciously feign symptoms in order to assume a sick role represent factitious disorder. Self-diagnosis of mental illness can facilitate validation and support from others, (eg, evoking sympathy and care from family, friends, teachers, and health care professionals). Self-diagnosis may also serve to avoid non-preferred tasks such as school attendance, homework, or chores. Psychiatric symptoms consciously faked to meet such a goal represent malingering. Symptoms produced unconsciously, often for unclear goals, represent a functional neurologic disorder.

SELF-DIAGNOSIS

Increasingly, young people go online to learn about and address mental illness. Recent studies found that 77% to 83% of youth surveyed would use the internet to find information or support for a mental health concern.[1,24] Many adolescents prefer to learn about mental health online because of easy, anonymous access to information. Although authoritative sources such as the American Academy of Pediatrics and the American Academy of Child and Adolescent Psychiatry have posted a wealth of free, reliable psychoeducation online, adolescents are increasingly likely to learn about mental illness via social media. Adolescents value learning about their peers' and admire influencers' opinions regarding mental health issues via social media, and often enjoy the entertaining (if extreme or inaccurate) way in which mental health information is presented on social media. Popular posts of mental illness on social media are typically rewarded with "likes" and followers, as well as a myriad of comments expressing support, caring, and encouragement, a fact not lost on adolescent viewers.

Mental health is among the most popular topics for TikTok and Instagram posts. At the time of writing the 16 billion TikTok posts with the designation #mentalhealth have been collectively viewed 140 billion times. Social media algorithms target specific demographics and audiences most likely to be interested in the subject matter, effectively disseminating information and awareness of mental health issues to groups not reached by traditional outreach methods. Algorithms favor posts which are engaging and/or entertaining over those which provide complete or accurate information, so popular presentations of mental illness are often extreme, and provide a skewed model for social learning. The popularity of mental health-related social media posts and limited verification or regulation of content combine to foster the spread of related misinformation. Social media influencers typically appear credible to youth because of their popularity, charisma, endorsements, and success despite the great majority lacking any related training or education. Content creators and non-medical social media influencers contribute to the dissemination of misinformation. Social media posts concerning mental health are typically misleading. One review of videos concerning ADHD on TikTok classified 52% as misleading,[25] while a study of 500 mental health advice videos on TikTok found 84% contained inaccuracies.

Mental health disorders are complex and influenced by a constellation of factors. Mental health providers rely on years of training and clinical experience to conduct a thorough interview, interpret mental status, compare collateral information, and often incorporate standardized interviews, assessments, and surveys to consider a broad differential before coming to a final diagnosis. Youth and parents self-diagnosing based on questionably trustworthy information from an online source, lacking impartial perspective, often results in misdiagnosis. Even trained medical professionals may misdiagnose based on familiarity and lack of objectivity, which is one reason the American Medical Association Code of Medical Ethics advises physicians against treating themselves or family members.[26]

It has become commonplace for patients and/or parents to present to health care providers requesting confirmation of a specific diagnosis and a particular treatment intervention. This situation puts providers in a difficult position, as those who disagree with the self-diagnosis risk damaging the provider-patient relationship and eroding trust. A patient who believes they have diagnosed themselves accurately may feel invalidated or misunderstood by a provider who disagrees. Self-diagnosis of a mental disorder may divert attention away from a proper evaluation for underlying medical problems. Patients who have misdiagnosed themselves often favor a specific treatment based on what they have discovered online, which may deter appropriate treatment, hinder recovery, and worsen prognosis.

Individuals may inadvertently over-report or under-report symptoms based on information available online, and may even unconsciously take on symptoms to which they are exposed. Youth may believe they have a mental illness when they do not, leading to unnecessary treatment, medications, and/or distress. On the other hand, some under-diagnose themselves, dismissing serious mental health issues that require professional intervention.

Youth who self-diagnose may attempt to manage their symptoms with ineffective or even harmful attempts at treatment based on misinformation or personal biases. For example, the "bed-rotting" trend on social media entails staying in bed during the day, binge-watching television, and using social media for hours or days in the name of self-care for depression. This practice runs counter to the accepted principles of behavioral activation, which recommends productive, active habits to address depression. Bed-rotting can impair sleep routines, displace physical exercise and activities of daily living, and paradoxically exacerbate depression. Some social media posts encourage or advise illicit substance use, eating disordered behavior, self-harm, and even suicide. Many easily accessed posts offer advice on how to carry these out, for example, how to conceal cutting behaviors from parents. Social media platforms' efforts to find and remove such posts are of limited effectiveness and are often evaded using coded language.

Social media can alleviate mental health stigma, but can also perpetuate stigma depending on content. The portrayal of mental illness on social media posts may contribute to misconceptions about mental illnesses, for example, that they are easily identifiable and self-treatable, or that people can simply "snap out of it." Self-diagnosis based on social media psychoeducation can conversely lead to feelings of helplessness or problematic justification of misbehaviors, for example, statements such as "I hit my peer because I am bipolar and can't help it" or "I can't do homework because I am depressed."

Should health care providers abandon social media? On the contrary, a need exists for accurate, useful psychoeducation, which providers are in a unique position to create. It is imperative for knowledgeable physicians and institutions to post positive content and to counter misinformation. Health professionals should advocate for social media companies, and the government, to recognize and address the potential for harm related to unverified mental health information available to youth online. It may be helpful to require disclaimers on posts making claims about mental health such as "I am not a health professional" or "this content is not a substitute for professional advice, diagnosis, or treatment" as indicated. Social media companies may emphasize content created by professionals, and that which focuses on wellbeing, prevention, treatment, and lifestyle interventions rather than romanticize pathology. Social media mental health posts could be required to clearly encourage viewers with questions to seek professional help and advice. Posts containing dangerous misinformation or encouraging eating disordered behaviors, self-harm, or suicide should be identified and removed, and repeat posters restricted.

CLINICAL VIGNETTE AND CLINICAL GUIDE

Sarah is an 11-year-old female, with no prior psychiatric history, who presents to the psychiatry outpatient clinic for an intake appointment. Her intake packet indicates she was referred by her primary care physician due to concerns for "inattention and difficulty socializing." Sarah states she would like to be treated for attention deficit hyperactivity disorder (ADHD) and autism. She reports her symptoms started in February 2021, during the coronavirus disease 2019 quarantine. She endorses inattention and restlessness in the school setting only. She also reports difficulties with falling and staying asleep, and has been staying awake at night to chat online with peers who live in another time zone. She has difficulty waking up in the morning, and sometimes naps in class. During class, Sarah often uses her cell phone to text friends or her school-issued computer to watch YouTube videos. She notes that she is good at multitasking and needs to watch a YouTube video to focus on the classwork. Sarah's academic functioning has declined. Previously an A-B student, currently she has a D grade average. She states that she has "ADHD paralysis," explains that sometimes her brain just "freezes" in the classroom and she cannot think. She states this often happens when she worries about being embarrassed or being judged by peers. Sarah reports being unable muster the courage to talk to peers "in real life (IRL)".

Sarah recently watched a TikTok influencer talk about their autism diagnosis, and identifies with their description of autism. Parent states that Sarah had always been a "social butterfly," but struggled socially for the first time upon return to in-person school in the Fall of 2021. She has since gravitated toward online relationships and refuses to engage in organized sports or extracurricular activities. At home, she has been able to do her chores and loves to keep her room organized. Regarding early developmental history, her parents do not endorse symptoms of an autism spectrum disorder.

During the visit, Sarah maintains good eye contact and engages in back-and-forth conversation. She states she feels "nervous at the moment" with an anxious affect. She sits calmly during the visit, however, is frequently distracted by notifications emanating from her cellphone.

QUESTIONS TO CONSIDER

The following questions can help guide clinical decision-making in cases like Sarah's:

- How do you broach the topic of self-diagnosis in youth?
- What are your thoughts about the differential diagnosis?
- How does the timeline and onset of symptoms lead to a working diagnosis?
- How does the presence or absence of core symptoms affect the final diagnosis?
- How does the self-diagnosis compare with your clinical diagnosis?

IN CLINICAL PRACTICE

The proportion of youth presenting to providers having self-diagnosed with a mental health condition (or having been diagnosed by a parent) appears to be increasing. Once a rarity, encountering an adolescent convinced they suffer from a specific psychiatric diagnosis has become commonplace. Informal polling of large groups of pediatricians and psychiatrists confirms this observation, and the authors' observations that the most commonly seen adolescent self-diagnoses include dissociative identity disorder (ie, multiple personality disorder), tic disorder, and autism. In the authors' experience, adolescent girls with limited in-person social support, who spend excessive time on social media, are most likely to self-diagnose. Youth who self-diagnose are often very invested in their diagnosis, for which they seek affirmation from providers and sometimes related treatment.

When a young patient presents with a self-diagnosis, a clinician's first step should be to assess concerns with a curious, open-minded approach.[27] This stance will help to build rapport and allows for the possibility that self-diagnosis may be accurate.

In the case vignette described earlier, a clinician could start by asking Sarah how she learned about her diagnosis and why she believes she has it. The use of open-ended questions will explore her subjective experiences, perspectives, and ideas freely. After the patient is able to tell their story, it becomes helpful to transition to more targeted questions. Providers should identify symptoms associated with suspected diagnoses and review related symptoms using criteria checklists obtained from the DSM-5-text revision.

Clinicians should ask what exacerbates and alleviates symptoms and determine how symptoms impact activities of daily living. For example, assessing the effect on sleep and school can provide invaluable information about behaviors that may worsen prognosis. It is helpful to inquire whether the patient has peers who suffer from the same condition, and how friends respond to the patient's difficulties. It can also be helpful to co-view a patient's social media feed (eg, TikTok's "For You" page) to assess the degree and nature of mental health content.

Collateral information is important for all psychiatric diagnoses of pediatric patients, but particularly critical in cases of self-diagnosis. Patients who self-diagnose may already be aware of related symptoms and readily endorse them, but it is vital to know whether teachers and parents observe them as well. Some level of disagreement in symptom constellation among these sources is typical, but significant disagreement should be explored and understood. When 2 sources agree but a third does not (ie, when a parent and child endorse symptoms of depression but teacher does not) it can be appropriate to give particular weight to the majority opinion.

In the case of Sarah, her self-diagnosis of ADHD should be explored by an interview with collateral contacts including her parents, teachers, and therapist if any. It seems likely that she is currently struggling with focus in class, but it is not clear that she had any such symptoms prior to the pandemic, as would be expected in ADHD. Furthermore, it is unclear if heavy screen media use is the cause of her poor attention in class, a contributor, or a response to it. It may be necessary to remove access to screens during class as possible to establish causality. Similarly, her insomnia may be caused by her screen media use in the bedroom, or vice versa. Restricting screen use in the bedroom at night for a reasonable period (ie, 1–2 weeks) can provide observable empirical evidence of causality. In both cases, if the problem resolves with screen restriction, no further treatment may be indicated. Sarah's self-diagnosis of autism seems unlikely given her parent's perspective that she does not suffer from related symptoms, and their memory of her as a "social butterfly" in childhood. Her own experience of her symptoms should be explored, as well as the perspective of her teachers, to help resolve discrepancies.

In cases in which a patient seems to have misdiagnosed themselves, it is important to understand the meaning and value the diagnosis has for them. The youth may be invested in a diagnosis to affiliate with a group of peers, online, or at school. Self-identification as mentally ill may arouse the interest or concern of peers, which can be reinforcing. The diagnosis may help them understand frustrations in their lives such as social, academic, or behavioral failures. It may explain and excuse misbehaviors or errors in judgment. Identification with a sick role may enable avoidance of non-preferred responsibilities such as going to school or doing homework (eg, by convincing parents that they are incapable).[14] Understanding needs that a misdiagnosis addresses in the life of a young person can help inform how to fulfill those needs in a healthier manner which does not require misidentification.

In cases where a provider determines that the patient has self-diagnosed incorrectly, it is our responsibility to inform the patient while respecting their perspective, autonomy, and experiences. Affirmation of a young person's ideas and feelings is important to maintaining therapeutic rapport, providing psychoeducation, and to facilitating ensuing collaboration. Validating a young patient's distress and concerns is important, especially in cases if the self-diagnosis is incorrect. If the self-diagnosis appears to help them meet a need, it may be helpful to problem-solve other ways that need could be met. For example, for a teen whose identification with bipolar disorder seems to connect her with peers who are interested or concerned, it may be helpful to connect her with other means of peer connection such as an afterschool activity or group therapy. For youth who appear to engage excessively with mental illness content on social media (especially if the content is triggering, makes them feel worse, or encourages unhealthy coping techniques like self-harm), it may be helpful for them to "block" such content from their feed to engage in more positive content. For youth who engage with social media excessively, it may be helpful to problem solve ways to limit social media to a healthy moderation and challenge the child to change their habits. Scheduled breaks from social media and rules which ban screens from the dinner table, the bedroom, at school, or during homework should be considered. In cases when a patient is unable or unwilling to moderate their use, parental restriction may be necessary. In extreme examples of toxic social media interactions or habits, complete internet restriction for a limited period may be necessary, while preparing for the possibility that doing so might provoke a crisis (eg, unsafe behavior) for youth who have become psychologically dependent.

RECOMMENDATIONS
For Caregivers

- Talk to your child about being skeptical about information they learn online, help them develop critical thinking skills.
- Educate your child about online misinformation, and teach them how to verify the source and the difference between professional experts and non-expert influencers.

- Children under 13 should be restricted from inappropriate content online including social media.
- Parents should regularly check the social media accounts of teens for their first year on social media and beyond if necessary, to monitor for inappropriate content and interactions, and be aware that youth may hide secret accounts.
- When youth are found to be engaging in inappropriate material via their social media feed or having unhealthy interactions online, parents should explain why these experiences are harmful and help their children to restrict unhealthy content from their feed and block contact with inappropriate individuals.
- Parents should maintain a structure in the home complete with limits on screen media use in order to foster a healthy balance of activities.

For Adolescents

- If you are concerned you may suffer from a mental health condition, discuss with your parent, caregiver, guardian, and/or a trusted adult (eg, teacher, coach, or pediatrician).
- Be aware of sources of misinformation online (eg, non-expert content creators, deep fakes, bots, online trolls) and how to verify and assess the source of online reports.
- If you are concerned about the health or safety of a peer, talk to an adult, and encourage your friend to seek professional help.
- Understand that psychiatric diagnoses made by oneself or one's peers are unreliable, and that following the advice learned on social media without the guidance of medical experts can be detrimental or even dangerous.

For Social Media Companies

- Posts making claims about psychiatric or medical conditions which are made by non-experts should be clearly identified for the viewer, along with a clear recommendation to seek consultation with a primary care provider or mental health professional if one is concerned they may suffer from a mental health condition or are thinking of self-harm.
- Posts encouraging unhealthy or dangerous behavior such as self-harm, eating disorder, or suicide should be effectively identified and removed.
- Improve algorithms to prioritize content that promotes mental health literacy and positive coping strategies, while minimizing the visibility of content that encourages self-diagnosis, romanticizes illness or self-harm, or perpetuates stigma.
- Allow users to easily flag posts that are concerning for mental health misinformation for review by the platform.

For Clinicians

- Educate patients on the prevalence of health misinformation on social media, and direct them to authoritative online sources to reliable sources such as the American Academy of Pediatrics (AAP) and the American Academy of Child and Adolescent Psychiatry (AACAP).
- Distribute authoritative handouts containing concise psychoeducation for patients with mental health concerns (eg, AACAP's Facts for Families).
- When a patient or their parent believes they suffer from a mental health condition, ask where they learned about the condition and perform an assessment, making sure to prioritize collateral sources of information (eg, teacher report).
- Ask patients about their social media habits and experiences, including what type of content they view or post about online.

- Invite patients who enjoy social media to share their social media page and posts with the provider.
- Educate patients who are engaging in mental health content on social media about the risks of doing so and help them block inappropriate or triggering content or contacts.
- Encourage a healthy balance between online and offline activities, including in-person socialization.

For Schools

- Children should receive thorough education on media literacy, how to assess the veracity of news reports and information they find online, and methods of source verification.
- Mental health curricula should include pitfalls of self-diagnosis, self-care, and caring for one's friends. Encourage students in need to seek help from adults, school counselors, and mental health providers.

SUMMARY

The way adolescents view the world and themselves is increasingly influenced by their social media experiences, for better and for worse. Understanding that many patients and their families now present for treatment bearing a set of ideas and expectations about their mental health and related needs, we must offer our own opinions and advice in a manner that adequately respects their preconceptions. It is our responsibility to help youth and their families develop a practical understanding of their health and wellbeing, and their ability to improve it, in doing so becoming alterative "influencers." Clinicians, particularly those who work with children, are role models and can be influential in their wellbeing.

CLINICS CARE POINTS

- Pediatricians should ask patients with mental health concerns and their parents what they believe about their situation and where they received this information.
- Pediatricians should warn youth and families about the risks of learning about mental health via social media and redirect them to reputable sources (eg, AACAP's Facts For Families available at www.aacap.org).
- Health care providers can support patients and caregivers by validating and investigating their concerns while coming to their own conclusion regarding diagnosis, understanding that self-diagnosis by youth and their parents is often unreliable.
- Pediatricians should ask youth and their parents what they believe the best treatment of their condition to be, and render their independent professional opinion, warning youth of the risks about learning about mental health solutions to be.

DISCLOSURE

The authors report no of conflicts of interest.

REFERENCES

1. Aboueid S, Liu RH, Desta BN, et al. The use of artificially intelligent self-diagnosing digital platforms by the general public: scoping review. JMIR Medical Informatics 2019;7(2):e13445.

2. Pretorius C, Chambers D, Cowan BR, et al. Young people seeking help online for mental health: cross-Sectional Survey study. JMIR Mental Health 2019;6(8):e13524.
3. Starvaggi I, Dierckman C, Lorenzo-Luaces L. Mental health misinformation on social media: review and future directions. Current Opinion in Psychology 2024;56: 101738.
4. Atske S. Teens and internet, device access fact sheet, 2024, Pew Research Center, Available at: https://www.pewresearch.org/internet/fact-sheet/teens-and-internet-device-access-fact-sheet/#: ~ :text=Today%2C%20nearly%20all%20U. S.%20teens,46%25. (Accessed 16 January 2024).
5. Rothwell BJ. Teens spend average of 4.8 hours on social media per day. Gallup.com, Available at: https://news.gallup.com/poll/512576/teens-spend-average-hours-social-media-per-day.aspx#: ~ :text=This%20use%20amounts%20to%20 4.8,for%2017%2Dyear%2Dolds, (Accessed 5 April 2024), 2024.
6. Little B. What prehistoric cave paintings reveal about early human life. HISTORY, Available at: https://www.history.com/news/prehistoric-cave-paintings-early-humans, (Accessed 5 April 2024), 2021.
7. Pierce WD, Bandura A. Social learning theory. Can J Sociol 1977;2(3):321.
8. Simply Psychology, Erikson's stages of development. Simply Psychology, Available at: https://www.simplypsychology.org/erik-erikson.html, (Accessed 5 April 2024), 2024.
9. Martínez V, Jiménez-Molina Á, Gerber MM. Social contagion, violence, and suicide among adolescents. Curr Opin Psychiatr 2023;36(3):237–42.
10. Giedd JN. Structural magnetic resonance imaging of the adolescent brain. Ann N Y Acad Sci 2004;1021(1):77–85.
11. APA dictionary of Psychology, Available at: https://dictionary.apa.org/social-contagion. (Accessed 5 April 2024).
12. Roback HB, Roback E, LaBarbera JD. Epidemic grieving at a birthday party: a case of mass hysteria. J Dev Behav Pediatr 1984;5(2):86–9.
13. Olvera C, Stebbins GT, Goetz CG, et al. TikTok Tics: a pandemic within a pandemic. Movement Disorders Clinical Practice 2021;8(8):1200–5.
14. Harness J, Getzen H. TikTok's sick-role subculture and what to do about it. J Am Acad Child Adolesc Psychiatry 2022;61(3):351–3.
15. Kramer ADI, Guillory JE, Hancock JT. Experimental evidence of massive-scale emotional contagion through social networks. Proc Natl Acad Sci USA 2014; 111(24):8788–90.
16. Fowler JH, Christakis NA. Dynamic spread of happiness in a large social network: longitudinal analysis over 20 years in the Framingham Heart Study. BMJ Br Med J (Clin Res Ed) 2008;337(dec04 2):a2338.
17. Samuels MA. Tik tok tics. Am J Med 2022;135(8):933–4.
18. Lewis SP, Seko Y. A double-edged sword: a review of benefits and risks of online nonsuicidal self-injury activities. J Clin Psychol 2016;72(3):249–62.
19. Swedo EA, Beauregard JL, De Fijter S, et al. Associations between social media and suicidal behaviors during a youth suicide cluster in Ohio. J Adolesc Health 2021;68(2):308–16.
20. Porter CA, Mayanil T, Gupta T, et al. #DID: the role of social media in the presentation of dissociative symptoms in adolescents. J Am Acad Child Adolesc Psychiatry 2024;63(2):101–4.
21. Littman L. Parent reports of adolescents and young adults perceived to show signs of a rapid onset of gender dysphoria. PLoS One 2018;13(8):e0202330.
22. American Psychiatric Association. Diagnostic and Statistical Manual of Mental Disorders. 5th edition. Arlington, VA: American Psychiatric Publishing; 2013.

23. Haltigan JD, Pringsheim TM, Rajkumar G. Social media as an incubator of personality and behavioral psychopathology: symptom and disorder authenticity or psychosomatic social contagion? Compr Psychiatr 2023;121:152362.

24. Dooley B, Fitzgerald A. Headstrong: The National Centre for Youth Mental Health. Dublin: Headstrong: The National Centre for Youth Mental Health; 2012. [2017 Oct 10]. My World Survey: National Study of Youth Mental Health in Ireland. Available at: http://www.ucd.ie/t4cms/MyWorldSurvey.pdf. Accessed April 5, 2024.

25. Yeung A, Ng E, Abi-Jaoude E. TikTok and attention-deficit/hyperactivity disorder: a cross-sectional study of social media content quality. The Canadian Journal of Psychiatry/Canadian Journal of Psychiatry 2022;67(12):899–906.

26. Riddick FA Jr. The Code of medical Ethics of the American medical association. Ochsner J 2003;5(2):6–10.

27. Weigle P. Psychoeducation or psychiatric contagion? Social media and self-diagnosis. Psychiatr Times 2023;40(5):14–5.

Social Media and Development of Sexual and Gender Identity in Adolescents

Daniel J. Suto, BS, MD[a],*, Jack L. Turban, MD[b], Erin L. Belfort, MD[c,d]

KEYWORDS

- Social media • Dating apps • Adolescents

KEY POINTS

- Social media offers adolescents alternative access to information, media, and relationships that facilitate key developmental tasks of gender and sexual identity formation and expression.
- For some youth, social media provides connection, support, and mental health benefits.
- Adolescents who form romantic relationships on social media also risk mental and physical harm, including worsened self-esteem, exploitation, abuse, or sexually transmitted infections and unwanted pregnancies.
- Although many adolescents are aware of these risks, clinicians should encourage risk-mitigation strategies, involvement of parental support, and referral to child psychiatry if indicated.

TERMINOLOGY AND BACKGROUND

This review aims to describe the current literature on the interplay between social media and gender and sexual development in adolescents. The authors use a developmental framework to describe the ways in which youth engage with social media as they navigate these developmental tasks. They offer a clinical vignette to highlight important themes and provide clinical tips for clinicians to assess gender and sexual development and their relationships with social media and online interactions.

Sexual orientation, gender identity, and gender expression are distinct concepts. Sexual orientation refers to the types of people toward whom one is sexually or romantically attracted. Gender identity refers to one's psychological understanding of their gender in relation to masculinity, femininity, a lack of either, or a combination of

a Department of Emergency Medicine, University of California, San Francisco, Zuckerberg San Francisco General Hospital, San Francisco, CA, USA; b Department of Psychiatry, University of California, San Francisco, San Francisco, CA, USA; c Department of Psychiatry, Maine Medical Center, Portland, Maine, USA; d Tufts University School of Medicine, Boston, MA, USA
* Corresponding author.
E-mail address: Daniel.suto@ucsf.edu

Pediatr Clin N Am 72 (2025) 279–289
https://doi.org/10.1016/j.pcl.2024.08.004
pediatric.theclinics.com
0031-3955/25/© 2024 Elsevier Inc. All rights are reserved, including those for text and data mining, AI training, and similar technologies.

both. Gender expression refers to the ways in which people present to the world in a gendered fashion through clothing, hairstyles, and pronoun use, among others. The term transgender will be used here as an umbrella term for individuals whose gender identities do not align with societal expectations based on their sex assigned at birth.[1] Transgender is used in opposition to the term cisgender, which refers to those whose gender identities align with societal expectations based on their sex assigned at birth. They also refer broadly to lesbian, gay, bisexual, transgender, queer, and other people that includes both sexual and gender minority (SGM) populations.

Importantly, gender identity development starts in the preschool years, prior to both social media use and the development of sexual identity.[2] Gender identity is a multidimensional construct that includes the relationship to gender roles and expectations, relationship to one's primary and secondary sex characteristics, and one's transcendent sense of gender. Research, including twin studies, suggests an innate biologic basis for gender identity.[3] Individuals build upon this innate scaffolding via language and conceptualizations of gender throughout development, impacted by one's family of origin, culture, and the larger sociopolitical context, toward a cohesive gender identity. Many establish a clear sense of their gender identity by early preschool years, while others continue to explore gender identity into adolescence and beyond.[4,5] By high school, an estimated 1.8% of youth now identify as transgender.[6]

The authors define sexual orientation as "a multidimensional construct that has been measured at least using 3 different dimensions: identity, behavior, and attraction."[7] Common sexual identities include heterosexual or straight (different-gender attraction), with sexual minorities including homosexual or gay/lesbian (same-gender attraction), bisexual (same-and-different gender attraction), and pansexual (attraction to all genders). SGM is an umbrella term commonly used to describe individuals who are not heterosexual and cisgender. Some academic and clinical literature focuses on action-focused categorizations, such as men who have sex with men (MSM) to highlight behavior over identity.

Sexual development is an important task of adolescence involving identity and intimacy. Traditional psychological theory by Erik Erikson highlights "Identity versus Role Confusion" and "Intimacy versus Isolation" as the primary developmental conflicts of adolescence and early adulthood, respectively.[8] Adolescence and young adulthood are characterized by the progression of sexual identity development, formation of intimate relationships, and identification with peers.[9] Erikson's stages are a theoretic framework; the underlying research of which was not conducted with consideration for SGM youth and therefore will not fully encapsulate the developmental tasks of SGM youth. In this review, the authors use the following developmental tasks to describe sexual and gender identity development of adolescents: identity exploration, formation, expression, community searching, intimacy exploration, autonomy, and risk taking.

The process of sexual development includes formation of sexual identity, sexual behavior, and intimacy. Cultural norms and expectations of sexual identity have significantly changed from the mid-20th century. The increased societal acceptance of sexual minority identities and increased representation of sexual minority characters in mainstream media exemplify this notable cultural shift. The Youth Risk Behavior Surveillance System (YRBSS), which tracks health-related behaviors of high school students with surveys every other year, provides the broadest contemporary dataset.[10] Overall, 88.8% of surveyed youth identified as heterosexual. Overall, 6% identified as bisexual. Overall, 2% identified as gay or lesbian. Overall, 3.2% were not sure of their sexual identity. Subgroup analysis by Philips and colleagues highlighted that

13.9% of female individuals assigned at birth and 7.0% of male individuals assigned at birth identified as Lesbian, Gay, Bisexual (LGB) or "not sure."

Sexual behavior is also described by the YRBSS.[10] For the years 2005 to 2015, 58.9% of youth had not had sex. The modal age of first sexual intercourse was 15 (11.2%). Among participants who had sex, the most common number of partners was 1 (16.5%) followed by 2 (7.8%) and 6 or more (6.0%). These data help contextualize an adolescent's sexual behavior. Several studies demonstrate overall decline of sexual behaviors among youth with resulting decreases in high-risk sexual behaviors and outcomes (eg, multiple sexual partners, sexually transmitted infections, and teen pregnancy).[11,12]

Sexual behavior still represents a somewhat taboo subject in American culture. The amount of sex education youth receive, if any, is highly variable, depending in part on differences in their families and educational environments. The Dutch model for sexual and gender education moves beyond preventative intervention or abstinence-only approaches to consider sexual health promotion interventions including considerations of pleasure, intimacy, and discovery. According to this model, healthy sexual behavior occurs in the context of a healthy relationship with one's body, positive self-esteem, clear consent, an understanding of potential outcomes of sexual behavior, and behavior that generally occurs in the context of a relationship.[13,14] One hypothesis offered to explain the decline in adolescent sexual behavior is the relationship with the release of the iPhone in 2007 and the swift uptick in youth having access to their own smartphones.[15] With the ability to connect via their device, in-person gathering, connection, and therefore sexual behaviors may have declined. Easy access to online pornography is also facilitated by smartphone use, and sexual gratification via pornography may have partially displaced interpersonal sexual behaviors.

For the purposes of this review, social media is defined as applications ("apps") or Web sites that facilitate communication between users (eg, through sharing messages, pictures, and videos). We use a broad definition that includes dating apps designed to connect individuals directly in addition to those who use an open platform. Social media use is very common among adolescents. The landscape of social media changes frequently as platforms rise and fall in popularity. In a 2022 study by the Pew Research Center, YouTube was the most commonly used platform with one large survey identifying that 95% of adolescents use YouTube, followed by TikTok (67%), Instagram (62%), and Snapchat (59%).[16] With the ease of accessibility to social media afforded by modern technology, many adolescents intertwine use with daily activities and some check hundreds of times per day. For example, of those who use TikTok, 16% are on the app "almost constantly."[16] Many social media platforms allow for either public or private user communication. Apps featuring video and image sharing can also facilitate social connection. In one survey, 41% of adolescents use social media to flirt.[17] Dating apps are also used by adolescents. Although many apps require users to be 18 years and older, age verification is lax. One study demonstrated that 19% of youth use dating apps while underage.[17] Dating apps can provide gender-specific and sexuality-specific spaces for connection, including geosocial networking apps, which allow users to share their locations in real time. SGM adolescents assigned male at birth frequently use dating apps. One study found that 60% of SGM adolescents who used geosocial networking apps had met someone from these apps in person.[18] Our discussion of why SGM youth use these apps, their potential risks, and how clinicians can speak with adolescents and families to address them can be found elsewhere.[19]

DEVELOPMENTAL TASKS OF ADOLESCENCE
Identity Exploration, Formation, and Expression

What is sexuality? What is gender? What can I be? Who am I?
Gender and sexual education in the United States is extremely variable among states, school districts, and families. As youth explore social media, they frequently encounter sexualized content. Youth often seek information about sex online, potentially building off sexual education received in schools or by families. Increasingly, social media has become a tool for sexual education.[20] SGM youth are often left out of cisgender heteronormative sex education conversations that occur in families or in health classes in school. This group of youth may be more likely to go online to seek health information and information about SGM identities and relationships. Mainstream acceptance of SGM people in media and in certain social media circles has made identity labels and identifiers more accessible to many adolescents.

Pornography (sexually explicit images or videos of people, with or without sexual behavior) is another common means of sexual exploration. The average age of first exposure to pornography in the United States is age 12.[21] Adolescent encounters with pornography are common and varied.[22] Reasons for pornography consumption among young people include in boredom, sexual gratification, to intensify masturbation, as means of exploring one's sexual self, and to learn about the mechanics of sex. Concerns that adolescent use of pornography may cause some degree of harm—including unrealistic sexual values and beliefs, reinforcement of highly gendered roles and sexual scripts, normalization of violent or coercive behaviors, and earlier experimentation—require further study.[23]

As sexual identity begins to form and solidify, sexual minority youth may choose to share their identity with others, commonly known as "coming out." Social media and online connections can serve as an important first venue for such identity expression. Online communities offer several advantages, including various degrees of anonymity and dedicated SGM communities. Relationships facilitated by social media can represent lower stakes settings for identity expression, particularly for adolescents who are not ready to share their identity with offline friends or family. Adolescents often feel more comfortable managing personal identity contextually (eg, practicing coming out in online spaces before doing so in real life).

Recent lay media have used the term "rapid-onset gender dysphoria" to refer to supposed maladaptive transgender identity development resulting from social media use.[24] This is not a validated mental health diagnosis, and the American Psychological Association has recommended against its use in diagnostic and clinical contexts.[25] Several lines of research provide evidence inconsistent with this construct.[4,24,26–29] Social reactions to gender identity—both peer and parent—are strong predictors of mental health outcomes for transgender and gender diverse youth, and clinicians should routinely assess a young person's social context as it relates to gender identity and sexual orientation. Clinicians and parents should ensure that adolescents are accessing information about gender identity from reputable resources and also screen for online and offline gender identity-related bullying victimization, which is sadly common among transgender youth.[29] Clinicians should also be aware of the broad range of gender identities and expressions among transgender youth and that not all transgender youth experience physical gender dysphoria or desire gender-affirming medical interventions. Those who do express a desire to better understand their gender identity or gender-affirming medical interventions should be connected with a therapist who specializes in these areas, as current guidelines require a comprehensive biopsychosocial mental health evaluation prior to accessing gender-affirming medical interventions for adolescents.[30]

Intimacy and Sexuality Exploration

Who can be a partner to me? What does intimacy look like? What does the expression of sexuality look like?

Relationships form on the basis of varying amounts of information shared, from anonymous chats to biographic profiles. As different platforms serve different purposes (text chat only, photo and video sharing, dating apps), requirements to self-identify and self-verify vary. Certain social media sites cater to specific goals of the user. For example, dating apps can provide more direct routes to intimacy than those focused on picture or information sharing. Dating platforms connect users one-on-one, in part by prompting users to identify what they are looking for casual sex, relationships, or even specific sexual acts.

Adolescents exploring intimacy and sexuality often use social media to flirt or send sexually explicit messages before attempting such communication in person. Such online exchanges, the first points of intimacy for many, may include messages describing sexual or romantic intentions, explicit sexual language, or shared photos or videos. The varying layers of anonymity offered by these apps encourage many adolescents to express vulnerability in a way they might avoid in person. Conversely, the possibility of those communications being shared by the receiver without the consent of the sender may inhibit others. Sexting has become a relatively normative experience among adolescents and will be explored in further detail in Englander and Weigle's study of this issue.

As social media can connect individuals across geographic boundaries, adolescents are able to form relationships across long distances. Free from the limitations inherent in relationships made at in-person venues (eg, school and neighborhood), adolescents can do so more selectively based on common interests, extended social networks, and specific romantic desires. This ability empowers adolescents to expand or diversify their social networks, particularly for those lacking social support in their immediate community.

Autonomy and Risk Taking

What does it mean to explore my desires? What are the consequences of sex? What is consent?

It is developmentally normative for adolescents to be curious about sexuality and explore intimacy and romance. Traditionally considered "adult" behavior, sexual exploration can be an exercise of autonomy. Familial and cultural expectations inform varying levels of stigma and perceived risk associated with sexual behaviors. Exploring adolescent autonomy often comes with risk-taking behaviors.

While social media platforms provide adolescents with more potential avenues for sexual and gender identity exploration, they are not without risk. Many of these platforms are designed for adults and fail to accommodate the unique developmental needs of youth. For example, researchers have identified alarmingly high rates of adolescent use of geosocial networking dating applications designed for adults.[18] There are inherent privacy and safety concerns for youth sharing their locations on these apps. Rates of sexual intercourse between people met via these platforms, including unprotected sex, are high.[18] Resulting relations between adults and minors may be inherently inappropriate or abusive.

In adolescence, bodily autonomy and understanding of consent can be impartially formed. Depending on cultural socialization, understanding of personal boundaries may or may not have been established by sexual education or by adult role models.

Clinicians and parents should advise adolescents regarding their bodily autonomy, their ability to consent for sex, and ways to maintain safety online. We have written advice on this elsewhere, specifically to reduce adolescent shame regarding online sexual behavior and encourage disclosure of potentially risky behaviors, to provide adolescents with developmentally appropriate spaces to explore gender and sexuality, and to counsel adolescents on relevant legal and social factors.[19]

PHYSICAL HEALTH RISKS

Incomplete sexual education often focuses on only highlighting the physical health risks of sexual activity in adolescents. As previously described, there are several developmental tasks associated with sexual exploration that are normative for adolescents. However, some sexual behaviors carry risks (eg, acquisition of sexually transmitted infection (STIs), unintended pregnancy, and intimate partner violence).

Research sheds light on the link between online behavior and offline sexual risk. One study found that adolescents who send more text messages are more likely to engage in risky sexual behaviors including condomless sex, sex without contraception, concomitant alcohol, and drug use.[31] This study identified correlation between online communication and offline sexual risk, but not causality between the two. Another study found that a minority of surveyed adolescents endorsed risky online sexual behavior (eg, searching for someone on the Internet with whom to talk about sex or have sex, sending photos/videos in which they were partly naked to someone they only knew online). Teens who engaged in risky online behavior were more likely to have had sexual intercourse with someone they had just met with or without protection. Predictive factors for risky behavior in this cohort included low educational level and high levels of sensation-seeking.[32] High-risk, and inherently abusive, situations can occur when adults have online relationships with youth. These interactions can lead to grooming, sex trafficking, and sexual coercion. It is essential to identify these relationships, establish safety plans, consider restricting Internet access, or even involving police or child protective services.

Most adolescents appear to be aware of the risks associated with such behavior. One study found that sexual minority male adolescents perceived risks to meeting partners from online venues including physical harm and deception.[33] Participants used various strategies to mitigate these risks: telling friends about plans to meet up with a partner, choosing a public meeting spot, and staying sober.[33] This literature suggests that counseling adolescents on risk-mitigation tactics may improve safety. It reinforces the need for developmentally appropriate safe spaces for SGM adolescents to meet others like themselves. Initiating non-shaming family conversations around gender and sexuality can be particularly helpful for SGM youth (eg, acceptance therapy).

MENTAL HEALTH RISKS

Social media has been linked, in pop culture and in research literature, to detrimental mental health effects in certain situations and populations. A frequently cited source of mental distress is the curation of a social media image that imparts unrealistic standards.[34] A young person's belief about the physical attributes and the lives of their peers are distorted from a myriad of technologic features, including filters and digital retouching of highly selected photo or video posts, posts selected to portray an idealized representation of self, and images that celebrate an "ideal" body image. Youth may perceive enormous pressure to post content that generates positive reactions from peers and may compulsively check social media for response to these posts or in response to a "fear of missing out," potentially worsening an experience of social isolation.

A sizable body of recent scientific inquiry investigates the effects of online relationships on mental health. One survey-based study found that adolescents endorsing high social support in online *and* offline settings had higher self-esteem, suggesting social media use may benefit this population. In contrast, those reporting high online social support, but low offline social support, had lower self esteem.[35] A study of adults found swipe-based dating app use to be associated with higher scores for distress, anxiety, and depression.[36] Participants with more extensive dating app use experienced greater distress and depression.[36] Paradoxically, participants believed that these dating apps improved their self-esteem.[36] Youth may struggle to accurately assessing impact of their own social media use. A Pew Research Center report found that most teens deny having good or bad experiences with social media themselves, but 32% believe other teens have mostly negative experiences.[37]

Interpersonal conflict between adolescents and online partners can impact mental health. Such conflict can include verbal abuse and manipulation. One study found digital dating abuse to be common among teens, especially girls.[38] The most frequently experienced abusive behaviors included digital monitoring and control (54%), direct aggression (46%), and sexual coercion (32%). These findings offer ample reason to screen for abusive online relationships among distressed teens.

Adolescents engaging in romantic or sexual interactions online frequently experience deception. The most serious manifestation is "catfishing," deliberately misrepresenting some or all of one's identity to further cultivate a relationship. Few studies have validated the impact of this practice on adolescents. One small study found that 65% of rural MSM had encountered deception on dating apps/social media sites, ranging from misrepresented dating interests, to fake or outdated photos, to entirely fabricated profiles.[39] Providers may share tactics to avoid deception with patients likely to seek romance online, including trying to verify identities, encouraging finding mutual connections with other friends, and video chatting before meeting in person.

CLINICAL VIGNETTE AND CLINICAL GUIDANCE

CLINICAL VIGNETTE

Emma is a 15 year old girl presenting for an annual adolescent clinic visit. She is otherwise healthy and has no acute concerns. A social history is obtained without parents in the room. Emma has been feeling sexual attraction to both boys and girls. She feels comfortable in her identity as a female. She denies dating currently but has been talking to JJ, a 16 year old girl she met via Instagram. JJ requested to follow Emma on this platform 6 months ago, and Emma accepted because they had a few mutual followers. Since then, they have been conversing more and more frequently, now messaging daily. They have bonded over their music tastes—Emma is considering meeting up with JJ at a concert next month. Since they do not go to the same school and Emma does not have a driver's license, they have not been able to meet in person before now. Emma is nervous but excited about meeting JJ in person. Emma is not sure what her parents would think about her going to this concert and she has not told them about JJ.

In this vignette, a routine social history elicits Emma sharing an online relationship that may become romantic. This situation offers an opportunity to encourage healthy relationships and exploration of sexuality, validate that interest in doing so is developmentally normative, and screen for unhealthy or unsafe behaviors.

The opportunity to screen for these unsafe online behaviors frequently presents to pediatricians, pediatric subspecialists as well as mental health providers. Commonly used mnemonics like the SSHADESS[40] framework (strengths, school, home, activities, drugs, emotions/eating, sexuality, safety) may reveal important information regarding social media use and online relationship formation. Direct, open-ended questions like "Do you meet people through social media?" may be more fruitful. Other validated tools to assess problematic online behavior have been published, however their use may not be necessary for all patients.[41] Using a curious, nonjudgmental tone when exploring these topics allows providers to validate adolescents while screening for unhealthy behaviors opening the door for nuanced discussions of social media use when appropriate.

Many clinicians caring for adolescents are comfortable screening for offline unhealthy and risk-taking behaviors. Extending this inquiry to online risk-taking behaviors is important to understand the vulnerabilities of the contemporary adolescent. Incorporating a social media history into routine social history inquiry and risk assessment may help foster a therapeutic relationship. The common digital divide between youth and adults allows teens an opportunity to act as an expert and to teach their clinician about social media apps in a health role reversal. Allowing teens to take this role may facilitate an understanding of how they explore developmental tasks in online spaces. Normalizing use of the Internet to explore intimacy and sexuality (eg, "a lot of teens have romantic relationships online") may allow youth to feel safe sharing these parts of their lives.

It is important to screen for sexual risks—both online and offline. Risky offline sexual behaviors or adverse outcomes include condomless sex, sexually transmitted infections, unwanted pregnancy, and coerced or nonconsensual sex. Risky online behaviors or adverse outcomes include sharing sexual images or videos, romantic involvement with adults posing as youth, grooming for trafficking or other forms of sexual victimization, and risks to privacy and personal safety when meeting potential partners in person. Mental and physical health risks of online behavior—as discussed previously—should also be screened for. This can include asking about self-esteem (Do you feel like social media makes you feel good or bad about yourself?), deception (When you are talking to someone you have met online, how do you make sure what they are saying is true?), meeting up offline (What ways are you protecting yourself if you decide to meet up with this person?), and abusive behaviors (Do you feel safe and supported by these relationships?).

Certain elements, discovered in history taking, might indicate a referral to child and adolescent psychiatrist or another qualified mental health professional. This includes evidence the adolescent meets criteria for a mental health disorder or engages in high-risk behaviors.

After gathering a social history, at-risk adolescents should be counseled on safest ways to use social media and explore relationships online. For example, Emma is exhibiting age appropriate behavior—she is exploring intimacy and relationships with others, exploring her identity and her sexuality, and discussing this appropriately with the practitioner. It is important to normalize this experience for Emma to prevent shame, which can preclude further discussions or lead to other mental health problems. Emma might be aware of the risks of meeting up with JJ, but it is unclear what steps she will take to protect her safety. She could be counseled to find ways to assure herself that JJ is not deceiving (catfishing) her by appropriate verification measures (eg, communicating on video chat, requesting identification). If she decides to meet up with JJ, she should consider meeting in public, bringing along a trusted adult, and staying sober during the meeting. She should be encouraged to identify means to reach out to if she feels unsafe at any point (including reaching out to a parent or the practitioner).

Emma has not told her parents about JJ. Nonjudgmental exploration could elicit her reasons, such as fear of sexual-minority stigma, rejection of online relationships, or familial/cultural beliefs discouraging sexuality and dating. Emma should be encouraged to discuss these topics with her family. The clinician may offer to facilitate these conversations to make them more comfortable. Adolescent confidentiality should be discussed with Emma, specifically that what she discloses is confidential unless there is a concern for harm to herself or others, including sex trafficking or sex work, abuse of minors or elders. If a provider suspects that a child may be a victim of sexual abuse, referral to child protective services is always indicated.

SUMMARY

Social media is a widely used and well-integrated part of everyday life for most adolescents. Teens use social media as a means to exercise developmental tasks of identity formation, intimacy exploration, and autonomy. Online romantic and sexual relationships have both potential risks and potential benefits that deserve nuanced discussions through this developmental lens. Given the near-ubiquitous impact of social media on adolescents, healthy and unhealthy behaviors and experiences should be screened at medical touchpoints when possible. If concerning behavior is elicited, physician counseling and possible referral to a child and adolescent psychiatrist should be offered.

CLINICS CARE POINTS

- Clinicians should screen for physical and mental health risks related to social media using nonjudgemental questions.
- Social media can offer developmentally appropriate relationships, including those for sexual and gender minorities.
- If concerning behavior is elicited, consider referral to child and adolescent psychiatry.

DISCLOSURE

None.

REFERENCES

1. Turban JL, Ehrensaft D. Research Review: gender identity in youth: treatment paradigms and controversies. JCPP (J Child Psychol Psychiatry) 2018;59(12): 1228–43.
2. Fast AA, Olson KR. Gender development in transgender preschool children. Child Dev 2018;89(2):620–37.
3. Diamond M. Transsexuality among twins: identity concordance, transition, rearing, and orientation. Int J Transgenderism 2013;14(1):24–38.
4. Turban JL, Dolotina B, Freitag TM, et al. Age of realization and disclosure of gender identity among transgender adults. J Adolesc Health 2023;72(6):852–9.
5. Gülgöz S, Glazier JJ, Enright EA, et al. Similarity in transgender and cisgender children's gender development. Proc Natl Acad Sci USA 2019;116(49):24480–5.
6. Johns MM, Lowry R, Andrzejewski J, et al. Transgender identity and experiences of violence victimization, substance use, suicide risk, and sexual risk behaviors among high school students — 19 states and large urban school districts,

2017. MMWR Morb Mortal Wkly Rep 2019;68. https://doi.org/10.15585/mmwr. mm6803a3.

7. Patterson JG, Jabson JM, Bowen DJ. Measuring sexual and gender minority populations in health surveillance. LGBT Health 2017;4(2):82–105.

8. Orenstein GA, Lewis L. Eriksons stages of psychosocial development. In: Stat-Pearls. StatPearls Publishing; 2023. Available at: http://www.ncbi.nlm.nih.gov/books/NBK556096/. Accessed December 3, 2023.

9. Christie D, Viner R. Adolescent development. BMJ 2005;330(7486):301–4.

10. YRBSS | Youth Risk Behavior Surveillance System | Data. Adolescent and school health. CDC; 2020. Available at: https://www.cdc.gov/healthyyouth/data/yrbs/index.htm. Accessed July 10, 2020.

11. YRBSS data summary & trends | DASH. CDC; 2023. Available at: https://www.cdc.gov/healthyyouth/data/yrbs/yrbs_data_summary_and_trends.htm. Accessed February 13, 2024.

12. About teen pregnancy. CDC; 2023. Available at: https://www.cdc.gov/teenpregnancy/about/index.htm3. Accessed February 13, 2024.

13. Schalet AT. Beyond abstinence and risk: a new paradigm for adolescent sexual health. Wom Health Issues 2011;21(3 Suppl):S5–7.

14. Naezer M, Rommes E, Jansen W. Empowerment through sex education? Rethinking paradoxical policies. Sex Education 2017;17(6):712–28.

15. Twenge JM, Park H. The decline in adult activities among U.S. Adolescents, 1976-2016. Child Dev 2019;90(2):638–54.

16. Vogels EA, Gells-Watnick R, Massarat N. Teens, social media and technology 2022. Pew research center: internet, science & tech. 2022. Available at: https://www.pewresearch.org/internet/2022/08/10/teens-social-media-and-technology-2022/. Accessed December 3, 2023.

17. Lykens J, Pilloton M, Silva C, et al. Google for sexual relationships: mixed-methods study on digital flirting and online dating among adolescent youth and young adults. JMIR Public Health and Surveillance 2019;5(2):e10695.

18. Macapagal K, Kraus A, Moskowitz DA, et al. Geosocial networking application use, characteristics of app-met sexual partners, and sexual behavior among sexual and gender minority adolescents assigned male at birth. J Sex Res 2019; 0(0):1–10.

19. Suto DJ, Macapagal K, Turban JL. Geosocial networking application use among sexual minority adolescents. J Am Acad Child Adolesc Psychiatry 2021;60(4): 429–31.

20. Todaro E, Silvaggi M, Aversa F, et al. Are Social Media a problem or a tool? New strategies for sexual education. Sexologies 2018;27(3):e67–70.

21. Watching Gender. How stereotypes in movies and on TV impact kids' development | common sense media. Available at: https://www.commonsensemedia.org/research/watching-gender-how-stereotypes-in-movies-and-on-tv-impact-kids-development. Accessed January 4, 2024.

22. Attwood F, Smith C, Barker M. 'I'm just curious and still exploring myself': young people and pornography. New Media Soc 2018;20(10):3738–59.

23. Owens E, Behun RJ, Manning J, et al. The impact of internet pornography on adolescents: a review of the research. Sex Addict Compulsivity 2012;19:99–122.

24. Turban JL, Dolotina B, Freitag TM, et al. Rapid-onset gender dysphoria is not a recognized mental health diagnosis. J Adolesc Health 2023;73(6):1163–4.

25. ROGD Statement. Coalition for the advancement & application of psychological science. Available at: https://www.caaps.co/rogd-statement. Accessed January 10, 2024.

26. Ashley F. A critical commentary on 'rapid-onset gender dysphoria'. Socio Rev 2020;68(4):779–99.
27. Restar AJ. Methodological critique of Littman's (2018) parental-respondents accounts of "rapid-onset gender dysphoria.". Arch Sex Behav 2020;49(1):61–6.
28. Bauer GR, Lawson ML, Metzger DL, Trans Youth CAN! Research Team. Do clinical data from transgender adolescents support the phenomenon of "rapid onset gender dysphoria". J Pediatr 2022;243:224–7.e2.
29. Turban JL, Dolotina B, King D, et al. Sex assigned at birth ratio among transgender and gender diverse adolescents in the United States. Pediatrics 2022; 150(3). e2022056567.
30. Coleman E, Radix AE, Bouman WP, et al. Standards of care for the health of transgender and gender diverse people, version 8. Int J Transgend Health 2022; 23(Suppl 1):S1–259.
31. Landry M, Turner M, Vyas A, et al. Social media and sexual behavior among adolescents: is there a link? JMIR Public Health and Surveillance 2017;3(2):e7149.
32. Baumgartner SE, Sumter SR, Peter J, et al. Identifying teens at risk: developmental pathways of online and offline sexual risk behavior. Pediatrics 2012; 130(6):e1489–96.
33. Jozsa K, Kraus A, Korpak AK, et al. "Safe behind my screen": adolescent sexual minority males' perceptions of safety and trustworthiness on geosocial and social networking apps. Arch Sex Behav 2021;50(7):2965–80.
34. Fardouly J, Vartanian LR. Social media and body image concerns: current research and future directions. Current Opinion in Psychology 2016;9:1–5.
35. Khan S, Gagné M, Yang L, et al. Exploring the relationship between adolescents' self-concept and their offline and online social worlds. Comput Hum Behav 2016; 55:940–5.
36. Holtzhausen N, Fitzgerald K, Thakur I, et al. Swipe-based dating applications use and its association with mental health outcomes: a cross-sectional study. BMC Psychol 2020;8. https://doi.org/10.1186/s40359-020-0373-1.
37. Rainie MA, Vogels EA, Perrin A. Creativity and drama: teen life on social media in 2022. Pew Research Center: Internet, Science Tech 2022. Available at: https://www.pewresearch.org/internet/2022/11/16/connection-creativity-and-drama-teen-life-on-social-media-in-2022/. Accessed February 13, 2024.
38. Reed LA, Tolman RM, Ward LM. Gender matters: experiences and consequences of digital dating abuse victimization in adolescent dating relationships. J Adolesc 2017;59:79–89.
39. Lauckner C, Truszczynski N, Lambert D, et al. "Catfishing," cyberbullying, and coercion: an exploration of the risks associated with dating app use among rural sexual minority males. J Gay Lesb Ment Health 2019;23(3):289–306.
40. Klein DA, Paradise SL, Landis CA. Screening and counseling adolescents and young adults: a framework for comprehensive care. Am Fam Physician 2020; 101(3):147–58.
41. Nereim C, Bickham D, Rich M. A primary care pediatrician's guide to assessing problematic interactive media use. Curr Opin Pediatr 2019;31(4):435.

Problematic Social Media Use or Social Media Addiction in Pediatric Populations

Carol Vidal, MD, PhD[a],*, Clifford Sussman, MD[b]

KEYWORDS

- Social media addiction • Problematic social media use • Behavioral addictions
- Prevention

KEY POINTS

- The design of social media platforms to keep users engaged creates inherently addictive platforms that can cause problems in younger ages.
- Research on problematic social media use is increasingly showing neurobiological, behavioral, and outcome-based similarities with substance use and other behavioral addictions.
- The evidence base on interventions for social media addiction is still nascent, but there is some promise shown by abstinence and reduction periods, as well as cognitive behavioral therapy.

INTRODUCTION

Social media (SM) facilitates social connections, information sharing, and entertainment. However, its use can become problematic. The negative consequences of SM at the population level are significant given its almost universal use. An estimated 4.9 billion people used SM worldwide in 2023, and the number of users is expected to increase to 5.8 billion by 2027.[1] In the United States, SM use grew from 5% of adults using at least one SM platform in 2005 to 50% in 2011%, and 72% in 2021.[2] Most users engage with SM at least once daily, about 39% admit feeling addicted, and 9% completely agree with the statement "I am addicted to social media."[3]

Over time, SM use has extended to all ages, and the age gap has narrowed. Yet, young people continue to use more than other age groups. There is a growing concern that developmental differences in habit-formation make SM's addictive power more noticeable among youth. In fact, national surveys show that 36% of adolescents

[a] Department of Psychiatry and Behavioral Sciences, Johns Hopkins University School of Medicine, 550 N. Broadway, Baltimore, MD 21205, USA; [b] Department of Psychiatry and Behavioral Health, George Washington University Medical School, Washington, DC, USA
* Corresponding author.
E-mail address: cvidal2@jhmi.edu
Twitter: @Carol_Psych (C.V.); @SussmancMd (C.S.)

Pediatr Clin N Am 72 (2025) 291–304
https://doi.org/10.1016/j.pcl.2024.08.005
0031-3955/25/© 2024 Elsevier Inc. All rights reserved, including those for text and data mining, AI training, and similar technologies.

pediatric.theclinics.com

say that they spend "too much" time on SM and 54% would find it hard to give it up, with most girls (58%) finding it especially difficult.[4]

The widespread commercialization of the smartphone in 2007 likely facilitated the reach and constant engagement on SM applications or "apps" to a level difficult to predict when Facebook first launched in 2005. Smartphones and SM apps have been adopted by increasingly younger individuals, with little use regulation. The coronavirus disease 2019 (COVID-19) pandemic was another turning point as shown by surveys of parents revealing an increased use of digital devices such as computers, smartphones, and game consoles, even in children aged younger than 11 years in 2021 compared to 2020. Furthermore, despite age restrictions requiring users to be at least 13 years old, SM use expanded across sites such as Facebook, Snapchat, Instagram,[2] with the largest increase being in "other" SM use (which doubled from 8% to 17%), and TikTok, which became popular during the pandemic and which use doubled from 13% in 2020 to 21% in 2021. Parents' concerns about children's screen time also increased.[4]

SOCIAL MEDIA USE AS AN ADDICTION

SM use that negatively affects personal, interpersonal, academic, and professional aspects of an individual's life has been described using terms such as "problematic SM use," "excessive SM use," or "SM addiction." While problematic Internet use was suggested as a disorder for the latest version of the Diagnostic and Statistical Manual of Mental Disorders,[5] the only disorder related to Internet use included under "conditions warranting further study" is Internet gaming disorder.[6]

There is controversy about whether behaviors in excess that are not related to the consumption of substances should be considered addictions. These "behavioral addictions" include pathologic behaviors related to gambling, food, sex, exercise, videogame and Internet use, and work. However, mounting biological and clinical evidence shows similarities and a need to address these behaviors, supporting the inclusion of behaviors such as pathologic gambling and Internet addiction in a category of "Addiction and Related Disorders."[7]

In the seminal article, "A 'components' model," Griffiths[8] advanced that behaviors could be considered addictions regardless of whether they involved the use of substances or not. Griffiths noted that specific common components to these behaviors included (1) Salience or the centrality of the behavior in a person's life; (2) Mood modification, or a feeling of calm or escape, and shifted mood when in need to cope with negative feelings; (3) Tolerance or the need to increase the frequency or amount of the behavior to achieve the same positive effect; (4) Withdrawal or the unpleasant psychological or physiologic feeling when the activity is discontinued or reduced; (5) Conflict, or the interpersonal and intrapsychic conflict, experienced by a person with addiction due to choosing short-term relief in exchange for long-term negative consequences; and (6) Relapse, or the tendency to repeat earlier behavioral patterns, often with a full reinstitution of the addictive behavior even after a long period of abstinence.

Both substance use and behavioral addictions are likely to have onset in adolescence, a period characterized by heightened risk-taking behaviors that increase vulnerability to the initiation and establishment of addiction patterns. In the case of substance use, earlier onset is associated with more psychosocial problems and substance use in adulthood. While evidence is still lacking for SM addiction, one would expect a similar pattern of worse psychosocial and clinical outcomes in adulthood with earlier onset of use.[9]

SOCIAL MEDIA FEATURES CONTRIBUTING TO ADDICTIVE BEHAVIORS

SM platforms' features make them potentially addictive. One aspect is the opportunity for social engagement linked to the behavior.[10,11] With SM, the drive to use may originate, or at least be maintained, by the need to sustain offline social connections and/or create new ones on the platform. This phenomenon comes at a time in human history of a certain degree of replacement of in-person interactions by technology. Yet, the innate need for human connection persists.

There may be differences in addictive potential by SM platform. For example, Nextdoor, a platform that facilitates communication with neighbors about events of interest, with geographic centeredness and potential for parallel in-person interactions, is qualitatively different from text-based platforms such as Twitter (X) or videobased platforms like TikTok, where the user interacts with people they may never see in person.

According to a study based on psychological and economic theories by Montag and colleagues,[12] the introduction of the smartphone created an "app" environment difficult to penetrate by scientists without the help of the app designers. The features of the phone apps and not the phone itself may be the culprit of the tendency to use in excess. The business model of Silicon Valley, where the user shares personal data instead of making financial payments, has the goal to keep the user engaged on the app for as long as possible, even to the detriment of other aspects of the user's life. These authors propose that a series of "app" features contribute to keep users engaged.

One feature with addictive power is the "endless scrolling and streaming" that facilitates the "flow," a state in which a person is so immersed with the task at hand that the perception of time is distorted. In SM, new videos or images appear without an automatic stop. At unpredictable times, the user sees content of interest or entertainment. This process follows an intermittent reinforcement schedule. As with slot machines,[13] a reward is delivered at irregular intervals, which seem random to users but are designed to keep them engaged. Intermittent reinforcement schedules are more successful than regular and predictable schedules of continuous reinforcement,[14] leading to the strongest type of behavior maintenance.[15] Most SM platforms have endless scrolling and streaming, and the user must make an active decision to disconnect from the "app." Notable platforms for endless scrolling and streaming include Instagram, YouTube, and TikTok where the next suggested video is selected for the user and previewed before the current video ends. TikTok's videos are typically 2 minutes or less (also referred to as "reels"). By shortening the length of the videos, the app incorporates yet another feature contributing to addictive behaviors: instant gratification. Soon after TikTok gained popularity during the COVID-19 pandemic, other SM sites, including YouTube and Snapchat adopted the characteristic "reels." Endless streaming also occurs with TV shows on the platform Netflix, which lead to show "binges," a behavior unknown to previous consumer generations whose only options were weekly sequenced episodes further interrupted by commercial breaks.

Another feature is the "endowment or mere exposure effect." This effect explains that the more time exposed to an online gaming world or effort expended building it, the more the user likes it and the harder it is to disengage from it. This feature applies to SM. In the case of Snapchat, for example, young people have "streaks," which are seemingly of no benefit to the user or the company, other than maintaining the user engaged. When 2 friends text back and forth frequently, they will have a longer "streak" or continuous days of texting. Once the user and a friend reach 100 days, an "emoji" (a digital icon to express an emotion or idea) appears next to the name of the user's friend. The "app" gives warnings if the streak is about to expire, which is after 24 hours of no engagement. In this process, a small action (eg, messaging a friend), becomes larger than the act itself, promoting daily app use.[16,17] This feature uses the exposure effect, along with social pressure. Montag and colleagues high-lighted the "double-tick function" in WhatsApp, a worldwide used messaging "app" that allows users to see if a message has been received and read. Younger genera-tions are now adopting colloquial language such as "leaving me on open" to signal when they know someone has read their message but has not responded.[18] Another addictive feature is the "Newsfeed" on Facebook, which shows the user's preferences and allows the company to track the user's product preferences and how much time they spend looking at them. TikTok is well-known for its strong algorithms that direct users to topics of their interest, providing endless user-created content.

SM provide many additional features with opportunities for social reward. Some ex-amples include the "like" on Facebook, the "love" on Instagram, and the former Twitter (current X)'s "retweet." Experimental studies of participants using Instagram have shown that more "likes," even when artificially controlled, have a stronger effect on brain areas related to reward processing such as the ventral striatum.[19,20] Social "apps" like Tinder, an online dating "app," require little effort to establish new interest relationships. Tinder also connects users geographically to people within their interest range. By swiping right or left depending on the user's interest, this app allows for im-mediate access to new social connections.

It is worth noting that not all negative effects of SM have been conceptualized under this model of addiction. Cognitive-behavioral principles can also help explain charac-teristics of SM problematic use such as the preference for online versus face-to-face social interactions and Internet use for mood regulation.[21]

EPIDEMIOLOGY OF PROBLEMATIC SOCIAL MEDIA USE

The global pooled prevalence of SM use in the general population nears 18%, with higher rates in the eastern Mediterranean region and in low/lower middle income countries. The increase in prevalence over the past 2 decades was exacerbated dur-ing the COVID-19 pandemic.[22]

A smaller sample of all SM users will experience problematic social media use (PSMU). A recent meta-analysis of SM addiction studies conducted across 32 coun-tries[23] showed heterogeneity in the prevalence, which ranged between 0% and 82%, depending on the threshold used to define PSMU. Studies with more conservative classifications for identifying PSMU had 5% prevalence, while those with the lowest threshold had a 25% prevalence. The authors noted that studies that use a lower threshold to define PSMU may be appropriate to guide prevention state-level and country-level policies, while studies with higher thresholds may be useful to guide clin-ical decisions about SM addiction.[23] An optimal threshold guide, for which more research is needed, would correspond to functional impairment. Interestingly, there are also cultural differences in SM use; collectivistic societies presented a higher prev-alence, likely due to the social pressures to conform to group norms of SM use.

NEUROBIOLOGY OF PROBLEMATIC SOCIAL MEDIA USE

Dopamine has been hypothesized as the main monoamine neurotransmitter involved in reward-guided behavior. Primates show greater tissue concentrations of dopamine and a peak of cortical dopaminergic innervation during adolescence. These neurobi-ological characteristics of adolescence parallel processes of autonomy from the caregiver, but may be associated with a higher risk for addictive behaviors in human adolescents.[24]

In substance use, a substance binds to receptors implicated in addictive behaviors. In behavioral addictions, changes in neurotransmitters are driven by the environment. Yet, both types of behaviors show similarities.[25–27] Structural and functional brain function changes with problematic SM indicate reductions in the volume of ventral striata, amygdala, and cortical areas, increases in ventral striata and precuneus activity (in response to SM cues), abnormal functional connectivity involving the dorsal attention network, and communication deficits between both hemispheres. These regions recruited with SM use are involved in the mentalizing network (perspective-taking and empathy), self-referential cognition (ability to relate information from the external world to oneself) and salience, reward, and the default mode network, also engaged in substance addictions. However, the small number of studies and heterogeneity of methods limit the strength of the conclusions. Well-powered longitudinal research is needed for a definite affirmation of corresponding processes between SM and substance use addictions.

PROBLEMATIC SOCIAL MEDIA USE AND MENTAL HEALTH

Most studies on PSMU focus on its relationship to mental health and behavioral problems. Systematic reviews and meta-analyses show SM use to be linked to depression and anxiety, suicidal thoughts and behaviors, poor sleep, body image, more distress, and poorer well-being.[28–33] There are only weak associations between time spent or intensity of SM use and mental health outcomes such as depression, but the associations between PSMU and depression are moderate. In children, time spent on SM, and especially PSMU, is both associated with depression, most notably in females, and with younger onset age.[34–36] Adolescents with attention-deficit hyperactivity disorder (ADHD) symptoms also present higher risk of PSMU than their peers without ADHD.[37] Other behavioral addictions such as Internet use, gaming, and gambling are risk factors for PSMU, but no associations with substance use treatment needs have been found.[38]

LIMITATIONS OF CURRENT RESEARCH

Existing research presents several limitations. First, there is a lack of agreement on the terminology. Many studies use *SM addiction*, while others use *problematic Internet or SM use*, with the intent to employ less stigmatizing language and avoid pathologizing the behavior. Second, many studies have used measures focused on one SM site (ie, Bergen Facebook Addiction Scale).[6,39] Given the rapid addition of new SM platforms, the development and use of scales that are applicable and sensitive to screen for all or at least some subtypes of SM are important.[40] The new Bergen SM Addiction Scale (6 items, public access)[39] is a good example of this transition. Another public access scale found to be acceptable is the SM Disorder Scale (9 items).[40,41] Finally, more research is needed to understand the differences between online and offline relationships.

CURRENT EVIDENCE ON THERAPEUTIC INTERVENTIONS

Universal approaches focused on screening and guidance are needed for all SM users. More targeted interventions for those at risk of presenting SM addictive behavior patterns can borrow from effective for substance use interventions such as motivational interviewing and cognitive behavioral therapy (CBT), assuming a similar model for substance use and SM addiction.

PREVENTION FOR THE GENERAL POPULATION

While SM can become an unhealthy habit manifesting addiction patterns and comorbidities that require moderation in its use, it also offers opportunities to increase communication, and access to entertainment and news from around the world. These advantages became vital in the context of the COVID-19 pandemic lockdowns, which limited activities outside the home. Considering the potential for addiction of psychoactive substances and other behaviors (ie,: video gaming and SM use), and the greater chances that these behaviors would be used for "escapism" and to alleviate pandemic-related stress, a group of experts provided guidance for healthy engagement with information and communications technology.[42] Their recommendations still apply after the pandemic and included (1) following daily routines and creating schedules that include work/study, socialization, and leisure time; (2) maintaining healthy sleep, eating, and personal hygiene habits; (3) exercising regularly; (4) using other stress-reduction techniques; (5) maintaining social connections, including with family; and (6) balancing news consumption: staying informed while limiting unnecessary exposure. More specific recommendations included self-monitoring one's screen time and reducing access to devices to self-regulate use; for parents, monitoring children's behavior, negotiating rules for use, being a good role model, and sharing some online activities with children to help them regulate their use; using digital well-being apps to limit time spent on SM and balancing it with screen-free time; and using analog tools when possible (ie, alarm clocks).

SPECIFIC INTERVENTIONS TARGETING PROBLEMATIC SOCIAL MEDIA USE

While the literature regarding the associations between PSMU and poor psychosocial outcomes is extensive, the research on SM-specific interventions is still scant.

In the general population, research following a model of addiction has examined SM use abstinence and reduction interventions with conflicting results. Some studies have found no benefits of SM abstinence. For example, a study examining loneliness, quality of life, and well-being found no differences between groups based on abstinence time (from 0 to 4 weeks).[43] Another study found differences based on type of use, with changes in affect among passive SM users (those who scroll and read other people's posts), but lower positive affect among active users (those who post and comment) after a 1 week abstinence period.[44] Other studies have found benefits of SM use abstinence and reduction. One study saw reductions in loneliness and depression in undergraduate students who limited SM use to 10 minutes per platform, per day, compared to a group using SM as usual.[45] Female adolescent dancers who abstained for 3 days showed reductions in body surveillance and body shame, and more positive mental states.[46] A group taking a week-long SM break presented improvements in well-being, depression, and anxiety compared to the group using SM as usual.[47] Another week-long trial found a 50% versus a 10% reduction in time spent on mobile SM to be beneficial to attentional performance and well-being, with decreased negative emotions in all participants, but no differences in outcome measures between groups. Abstaining from Facebook for 5 days was also associated with lower levels of cortisol and life satisfaction than continuing to use as usual.[48] However, participants may be substituting SM with other forms of technology (ie, video games). Future research will need to explore differences between all-technology abstinence and SM-only abstinence.

Beyond abstinence and reduction studies, there is potential for improved affect with interventions on cognitive mechanisms related to social comparisons. Experimental studies with Romanian high schoolers who were asked to compare downwards (with others who are worse off) showed increased gratitude.[49] In college students, a self-help intervention (combined CBT with cognitive reconstruction about SM use) reduced PSMU and improved mental health and academic outcomes.[50] The intervention included daily diaries with reflections and reminder cards about a reflection on the advantages of reducing SM use and the disadvantages of excessive use as a phone lock screen. Finally, therapy-based interventions appear to be more effective in improving mental well-being than abstinence-based and use reduction interventions, the latter of which are the least effective.[51]

Combining approaches may also be beneficial. Integrating CBT, short abstinence periods, and daily dairies over a 2 week period showed improved life satisfaction compared to daily diaries and SM use as usual.[52] The support for CBT interventions for SM is drawn mostly from literature on Internet addiction.[53–56] There is certain overlap between Internet and SM addiction. Half of US teens spend 4.8 hours daily on SM on average,[57] suggesting that much of the time spent on screens is used to navigate SM sites. However, SM-specific interventions are understudied.[58] Parental restrictions may be beneficial in decreasing time spent on SM, suggesting a role of family therapy, which has proven effective for Internet addiction.[59,60]

WHAT CAN WE LEARN FROM OTHER BEHAVIORAL ADDICTIVE DISORDERS INTERVENTIONS?

Adapted interventions common in substance use disorders may have a role in technology addictions. Research on addictive behaviors on digital technologies (ie, Internet, smartphones, and computers), such as on-line games, pornography, and shopping addictions, is advanced[11,61] and includes adolescents and young adults.[11] Notably, activities such as Internet-based massive multiplayer gaming with built-in chat features are becoming increasingly social, and more difficult to distinguish from SM.

The literature supports CBT,[62] Acceptance and Cognitive Restructuring, and Craving Behavioral Interventions as promising interventions for gaming disorder.[63] However, the studies conducted on CBT did not include PSMU scales. Other propitious treatments include motivational interviewing, mindfulness, exercise, and family-based interventions.[64–68] Regarding medications, one open label study suggested antidepressants as potentially useful in treating Internet addiction.[69] A recent review on psychopharmacological interventions for all technological addictions showed supporting evidence for the use of stimulants (ie, methylphenidate), antidepressants (ie, escitalopram and bupropion)[70] and CBT for Internet gaming disorder, and CBT as a valid treatment for SM addiction, online porn, and shopping addictions.[71] Bupropion, an antidepressant medication with dopaminergic and noradrenergic properties, is effective for Internet gaming disorder treatment independently of the presence of comorbid depression.[72] As with other disorders of addiction and mental health, combined psychosocial and pharmacologic interventions seem to be more effective for Internet use disorders than either approach alone.[73]

DISCUSSION

Based on existing research, addressing PSMU requires multilevel interventions.

Policy

Broad-level interventions involve federal-level and state-level restrictions on youth's access to SM platforms and their addictive features. While important, the ubiquitous presence, use, and constant evolution of SM make regulation challenging. Public health campaigns explaining the risks for addiction at a young age and the ways to manage SM use could be used for public education. Guidance by the medical and educational communities on the appropriate age for smartphone acquisition and exposure to SM is needed. However, individual differences among children should be considered. The US Congress and some states have already enacted laws to protect children and prevent excessive or early SM access. Clinicians should continue to be part of these conversations.

School/Community

Some schools across the country have enacted policies to limit cell phone use in the building or during class. School interventions to limit screen-based entertainment have potential for positive effects on student academic and behavioral outcomes. Support by parents (ie, to restricting smartphone use in school) should be addressed educating communities about the risks of SM use.

Schools also have a role in educating children about SM's potential negative effects, including its addictive nature. Teaching good habit formation and healthy use of SM could provide students with the skills necessary to self-regulate their use. Schools can also promote digital media citizenship, teaching students safe and responsible ways to interact with each other online.

The trend in schools to heavily rely on technology in the classroom needs to be discussed in the context of screen addictions. Appropriate use of technology can optimize educational outcomes,[74,75] but there are risks such as distraction, technology misuse during school hours, and disruption of efforts to regulate healthy screen use at home with school-issued technology and digital assignments. Technology use to complement and not substitute traditional teaching methods may be most beneficial. Options for individual accommodations for those struggling with PSMU, such as paper-based assignments and additional monitoring of technology use during class time can be helpful.

Clinicians

Professional associations should update guidelines on screen time limits to include SM use, given the changing environment that has left previous guidelines outdated. Clinicians working with children should consider including Internet-related behavior (including SM use) as part of their assessments. Helping families set screen limits and understand the risks of problematic SM, and brief interventions with aspects of healthy-habit building, motivational interviewing, and CBT can be beneficial and feasible in pediatrician's offices. If screening questions identify that SM is negatively impacting overall health (ie, displacing sleep, exercise, and nutrition) or mental health (ie, impaired self-esteem, depression, and anxiety), referral to a psychiatrist and/or psychotherapist may be helpful. In cases with severe symptoms such as school avoidance or suicidality, placement in a psychiatric hospital, residential center, or other specialized program may be warranted.

Families

As consensus on what is healthy SM use and regulation remains challenging, much of the burden for safely navigating a world overrun with SM falls to the home environment. Families can help shape behaviors by instilling healthy routines, off-screen activities, and better placement of cues (ie, keeping digital devices in a different location from schoolwork and sleep areas). Parents or guardians may also add structure, such as programming of outdoor activities and regular exercise, helping children navigate unstructured time with time-limited blocks of SM use, and delaying the age of acquiring smartphones. Parents can model by moderating their own use, eliminating smartphone use at mealtimes, and scheduling in-person social activities, which can positively affect the entire family's SM use habits. Family media plans can be created with online resources. Parents should seek professional help when their children show signs of addiction. Future research should focus on the effectiveness of periods of brief abstinence from digital devices as a family intervention.

Individuals

Children can learn to schedule their SM use, avoiding use at night or early in the morning, and prioritizing other activities, such as school work, sports, and face-to-face time with friends and family. Young adults may need support after leaving home onto more unstructured or unsupervised environments.

SUMMARY

The current universal use of SM among children places them at risk for SM addictive behaviors. Pediatricians already provide guidance for healthy-behavior formation and can incorporate SM use screening and guidance in their practices. While the research on effective interventions specific to SM use is still growing, brief periods of abstinence, family media plans, and an overall mindful use of technology that promotes other health-related behaviors such as sleep and in-person socialization may benefit children's development. More severe addictive behaviors or other mental health comorbidities may require referral to mental health specialists.

CLINICS CARE POINTS

- SM use is now almost universal among youth, and a proportion of children will develop addictive use patterns on these platforms.
- Children can learn to schedule their SM use, avoiding use at night or early in the morning, and prioritizing activities such as school work, sports and in-person interactions.
- Pediatricians can involve families and provide anticipatory guidance, promoting healthy behaviors, screening for PSMU, providing brief interventions, and referring to specialists as needed.
- Brief interventions with aspects of healthy-habit building, motivational interviewing, and CBT can be beneficial. Brief abstinence, use reduction and periods of self-monitoring show promise.
- For children with acute dysfunction related to SM use, additional interventions and referral to a psychiatrist and/or psychotherapist should be considered.
- In case of severe symptoms such as school avoidance or suicidality, psychiatric placement may be warranted.

DISCLOSURE

The authors have no commercial or financial conflicts of interest. Funding: Dr C. Vidal currently receives research grant funding from the Maryland Department of Health,

United States, and the American Academy of Child & Adolescent Psychiatry, United States, and the National Institute on Drug Abuse, United States of the National Institutes of Health (Physician Scientist Career Development Award [K12DA000357]). The content is solely the responsibility of the authors and does not necessarily represent the official views of the National Institutes of Health.

REFERENCES

1. Wong B. and Bottorff C., Top social media Statistics and trends of 2024. Forbes Advisor Web site, Available at: https://www.forbes.com/advisor/business/social-media-statistics/#source, (Accessed 4 August 2024), 2023.
2. Pew Research Center. Social media fact sheet. Fact sheets: tech adoption trends. 2021.
3. ThinkNow. Share of online users in the United States who report being addicted to social media as of April 2019, by age group. 2019. Available at: https://www.statista.com/statistics/1081292/social-media-addiction-by-age-usa/. Accessed January 31, 2024.
4. Vogels EA, Gelles-Watnick R. Teens and social media: key findings from pew research center surveys. Pew research center web site. 2023. Available at: https://www.pewresearch.org/short-reads/2023/04/24/teens-and-social-media-key-findings-from-pew-research-center-surveys/. Accessed January 31, 2024.
5. American Psychiatric Association, American Psychiatric Association. DSM-5 Task Force. Diagnostic and statistical manual of mental disorders : DSM-5. 5th edition. Arlington, VA: American Psychiatric Publishing; 2013.
6. Bányai F, Zsila Á, Király O, et al. Problematic social media use: results from a large-scale nationally representative adolescent sample. PLoS One 2017;12(1): e0169839.
7. Grant JE, Potenza MN, Weinstein A, et al. Introduction to behavioral addictions. Am J Drug Alcohol Abuse 2010;36(5):233–41.
8. Griffiths M. A 'components' model of addiction within a biopsychosocial framework. J Subst Use 2005;10(4):191–7.
9. Vidal C, Meshi D. Behavioral addictive disorders in children and adolescents. J Am Acad Child Adolesc Psychiatry 2023;62(5):512–4.
10. Griffiths MD, Kuss DJ, Demetrovics Z. Chapter 6 - social networking addiction: an overview of preliminary findings. Cambridge, MA: Behavioral AddictionsElsevier Inc; 2014. p. 119–41.
11. Sussman CJ, Harper JM, Stahl JL, et al. Internet and video game addictions: diagnosis. Epidemiol Neurobiol 2018;27(2):307–26.
12. Montag C, Lachmann B, Herrlich M, et al. Addictive features of social media/messenger platforms and freemium games against the background of psychological and economic theories. Int J Environ Res Publ Health 2019;16(14):2612.
13. Harrigan KA, Dixon M, Sheets PAR. probabilities, and slot machine play: implications for problem and non-problem gambling. J Gambl Stud 2009;(23):81.
14. Ferster CB, Skinner BF. Schedules of reinforcement. New York, NY: Appleton; 1957.
15. Tarbox J, Tarbox C. Training Manual for Behavior Technicians Working with Individuals with Autism. In: Training Manual for Behavior Technicians Working with Individuals with Autism. Cambridge, MA: Academic Press; 2017. p. 47–87.
16. Snapchat. How do Snapstreaks work and when do they expire?. Available at: https://help.snapchat.com/hc/en-us/articles/7012394193684-How-do-Snapstreaks-work-and-when-do-they-expire. Accessed January 31, 2024.

17. William Antonelli, edited by John Lynch. How to start a Snapchat streak and keep it alive to boost your Snap score. Business insider web site. Available at: https://www.businessinsider.com/guides/tech/snapchat-streak. Accessed January 31, 2024.

18. Left on open. Urban dictionary web site. Available at: https://www.urbandictionary.com/. Accessed January 31, 2024.

19. Sherman LE, Payton AA, Hernandez LM, et al. The power of the like in adolescence: effects of peer influence on neural and behavioral responses to social media. Psychol Sci 2016;27(7):1027–35.

20. Sherman LE, Greenfield PM, Hernandez LM, et al. Peer influence via Instagram: effects on brain and behavior in adolescence and young adulthood. Child Dev 2018;89(1):37–47.

21. Varona MN, Muela A, Machimbarrena JM. Problematic use or addiction? A scoping review on conceptual and operational definitions of negative social networking sites use in adolescents. Addict Behav 2022;134:107400.

22. Meng S, Cheng J, Li Y, et al. Global prevalence of digital addiction in general population: a systematic review and meta-analysis. Clin Psychol Rev 2022;92:102128.

23. Cheng C, Lau Y, Chan L, et al. Prevalence of social media addiction across 32 nations: meta-analysis with subgroup analysis of classification schemes and cultural values. Addict Behav 2021;117:106845.

24. Enns A, Orpana H. Original quantitative research - autonomy, competence and relatedness and cannabis and alcohol use among youth in Canada: a cross-sectional analysis. Health Promot Chronic Dis Prev Can 2020;40(5–6):201–10.

25. He Q, Turel O, Bechara A. Brain anatomy alterations associated with Social Networking Site (SNS) addiction. Sci Rep 2017;7(1):45064.

26. He Q, Turel O, Bechara A. Association of excessive social media use with abnormal white matter integrity of the corpus callosum. Psychiatry Res Neuroimaging 2018;278:42–7.

27. Turel O, He Q, Brevers D, et al. Social networking sites use and the morphology of a social-semantic brain network. Soc Neurosci 2018;13(5):628–36.

28. Lopes LS, Valentini JP, Monteiro TH, et al. Problematic social media use and its relationship with depression or anxiety: a systematic review. Cyberpsychol Behav Soc Netw 2022;25(11):691–702.

29. Huang C. A meta-analysis of the problematic social media use and mental health. Int J Soc Psychiatry 2022;68(1):12–33.

30. Alonzo R, Hussain J, Stranges S, et al. Interplay between social media use, sleep quality, and mental health in youth: a systematic review. Sleep Med Rev 2021;56:101414.

31. Nesi J, Burke TA, Bettis AH, et al. Social media use and self-injurious thoughts and behaviors: a systematic review and meta-analysis. Clin Psychol Rev 2021;87:102038.

32. Shannon H, Bush K, Villeneuve PJ, et al. Problematic social media use in adolescents and young adults: systematic review and meta-analysis. JMIR Ment Health 2022;9(4):e33450.

33. Bozzola E, Spina G, Agostiniani R, et al. The use of social media in children and adolescents: Scoping Review on the Potential Risks. Int J Environ Res Public Health 2022;19(16):9960.

34. Cunningham S, Hudson CC, Harkness K. Social media and depression symptoms: a meta-analysis. Res Child Adolesc Psychopathol 2021;49(2):241–53.

35. Vidal C, Lhaksampa T, Miller L, et al. Social media use and depression in adolescents: a scoping review. Int Rev Psychiatry 2020;32(3):235–53.

36. Hussain Z, Griffiths MD. Problematic social networking site use and comorbid psychiatric disorders: a systematic review of recent large-scale studies. Front Psychiatry 2018;9:686.

37. Dekkers TJ, van Hoorn J. Understanding problematic social media use in adolescents with attention-deficit/hyperactivity disorder (ADHD): a narrative review and clinical recommendations. Brain Sci 2022;12(12):1625.

38. Henzel V, Håkansson A. Hooked on virtual social life. Problematic social media use and associations with mental distress and addictive disorders. PLoS One 2021;16(4):e0248406.

39. Andreassen CS, Torsheim T, Brunborg GS, et al. Development of a. Facebook Addiction Scale 2012;110(2):501.

40. van den Eijnden RJJM, Lemmens JS, Valkenburg PM. The Social Media Disorder Scale. Comput Hum Behav 2016;61:478–87.

41. Schlossarek S, Schmidt H, Bischof A, et al. Psychometric properties of screening instruments for social network use disorder in children and adolescents: a systematic review. JAMA Pediatr 2023;177(4):419–26.

42. Király O, Potenza MN, Stein DJ, et al. Preventing problematic internet use during the COVID-19 pandemic: consensus guidance. Compr Psychiatry 2020;100: 152180.

43. Hall JA, Xing C, Ross EM, Johnson RM. Experimentally manipulating social media abstinence: results of a four-week diary study. Media Psychol 2021;24(2):259–75.

44. Hanley SM, Watt SE, Coventry W. Taking a break: the effect of taking a vacation from Facebook and Instagram on subjective well-being. PLoS One 2019;14(6): e0217743.

45. Hunt MG, Marx R, Lipson C, et al. No more FOMO: limiting social media decreases loneliness and depression 2018;37(10):751–68.

46. Roberts T, Daniels EA, Weaver JM, et al. "Intermission!" A short-term social media fast reduces self-objectification among pre-teen and teen dancers. Body Image 2022;43:125–33.

47. Lambert J, Barnstable G, Minter E, et al. Taking a one-week break from social media improves well-being, depression, and anxiety: a randomized controlled trial. Cyberpsychol, Behav Soc Netw 2022;25(5):287–93.

48. Vanman EJ, Baker R, Tobin SJ. The burden of online friends: the effects of giving up Facebook on stress and well-being. J Soc Psychol 2018;158(4):496–508.

49. Nicuţă EG, Constantin T. Take nothing for granted: downward social comparison and counterfactual thinking increase adolescents' state gratitude for the little things in life. J Happiness Stud 2021;22(8):3543–70.

50. Hou Y, Xiong D, Jiang T, et al. Social media addiction: its impact, mediation, and intervention. Cyberpsychology 2019;13(1).

51. Plackett R, Blyth A, Schartau P. The impact of social media use interventions on mental well-being: systematic review. J Med Internet Res 2023;25(4):e44922.

52. Zhou X, Rau PP, Yang C, et al. Cognitive behavioral therapy-based short-term abstinence intervention for problematic social media use: improved well-being and underlying mechanisms. Psychiatr Q 2021;92(2):761–79.

53. Weinstein A, Curtiss Feder L, Rosenberg KP, et al. Internet addiction disorder. In: internet addiction disorder. In: Rosenberg KP, Curtiss Feder L, editors. Behavioral Addiction. Cambridge, MA: Elsevier Academic Press; 2014. p. 99–117.

54. Pontes HM, Kuss DJ, Griffiths M. Clinical psychology of Internet addiction: a review of its conceptualization, prevalence, neuronal processes, and implications for treatment. Dove Press J 2015;(4):11–23.

55. Wölfling K, Beutel ME, Dreier M, et al. Treatment outcomes in patients with internet addiction: a clinical pilot study on the effects of a cognitive-behavioral therapy program. BioMed Res Int 2014;2014:425924–8.

56. Zajac K, Ginley MK, Chang R, et al. Treatments for internet gaming disorder and internet addiction: a systematic review. Psychol Addict Behav 2017;31(8): 979–94.

57. Rothwell J. How parenting and self-control mediate the link between social media use and youth mental health . Institute of family studies web site. 2023. Available at: https://ifstudies.org/blog/how-parenting-and-self-control-mediate-the-link-between-social-media-use-and-youth-mental-health. Accessed January 31, 2024.

58. Rothwell J. Gallup: teens spend average of 4.8 hours on social media per day. Washington, DC: Targeted News Service; 2023.

59. Liu Q, Fang X, Yan N, et al. Multi-family group therapy for adolescent Internet addiction: exploring the underlying mechanisms. Addict Behav 2015;42:1–8.

60. Dtl S, Tang V, Cy L. Evaluation of an internet addiction treatment program for Chinese adolescents in Hong Kong. Adolescence 2009;44(174):359–73.

61. Greenfield DN. Psychological characteristics of compulsive internet use: a preliminary analysis. Cyberpsychol Behav 1999;2(5):403–12.

62. Stevens MWR, King DL, Dorstyn D, et al. Cognitive–behavioral therapy for Internet gaming disorder: a systematic review and meta-analysis. Clin Psychol Psychother 2019;26(2):191–203.

63. Chen Y, Lu J, Wang+ L, Gao X. Effective interventions for gaming disorder: a systematic review of randomized control trials. Front Psychiatry 2023;14:1098922.

64. Xu L, Wu L, Geng X, et al. A review of psychological interventions for internet addiction. Psychiatry Res 2021;302:114016.

65. Schmidt H, Brandt D, Meyer C, et al. Motivational brief interventions for adolescents and young adults with Internet use disorders: a randomized-controlled trial. J Behav Addict 2022;11(3):754–65.

66. Bottel L, Brand M, Dieris-Hirche J, Herpertz S, Timmesfeld N, Te Wildt BT. Efficacy of short-term telemedicine motivation-based intervention for individuals with Internet Use Disorder – a pilot-study. J Behav Addict 2021;10(4):1005–14.

67. Bonnaire C, Liddle HA, Har A, Nielsen P, Phan O. Why and how to include parents in the treatment of adolescents presenting Internet gaming disorder? J Behav Addict 2019;8(2):201–12.

68. Zhang X, Yang H, Zhang K, et al. Effects of exercise or tai chi on Internet addiction in college students and the potential role of gut microbiota: a randomized controlled trial. J Affect Disord 2023;327:404–15.

69. Dell'osso B, Hadley S, Allen A, Baker B, Chaplin Wf, Hollander E. Escitalopram in the treatment of impulsive-compulsive internet usage disorder : an open-label trial followed by a double-blind discontinuation phase. J Clin Psychiatry 2008; 69(3):452–6.

70. Song J, Park JH, Han DH, et al. Comparative study of the effects of bupropion and escitalopram on Internet gaming disorder. Psychiatry Clin Neurosci 2016; 70(11):527–35.

71. Sherer J, Levounis P. Technological addictions. Psychiatr Clin North Am 2022; 45(3):577–91.

72. Seo EH, Yang H, Kim S, Park S, Lee S, Yoon H. A literature review on the efficacy and related neural effects of pharmacological and psychosocial treatments in individuals with internet gaming disorder. Psychiatry Investig 2021;18(12):1149–63.

73. Chang C, Chang Y, Yang L, Tzang R. The comparative efficacy of treatments for children and young adults with internet addiction/internet gaming disorder: an updated meta-analysis. Int J Environ Res Public Health 2022;19(5):2612.

74. Zheng B, Warschauer M, Lin C, Chang C. Learning in one-to-one laptop environments: a meta-analysis and research synthesis. Rev Educ Res 2016;86(4):1052–84.

75. Simões S, Oliveira T, Nunes C. Influence of computers in students' academic achievement. Heliyon 2022;8(3):e09004.

Social Media and Youth Well-Being

Considerations for Historically, Persistently, and Systemically Marginalized Groups

Seeba Anam, MD[a],*, Jane Harness, DO[b]

KEYWORDS

- Social media • Youth • Mental health • Legal • Caregiver • Discrimination

KEY POINTS

- Social media use has unique contributions to both ill-being and well-being for youth.
- Social media usage may vary by developmental age and group, which contextualizes its impact.
- Recommendations about social media use should be tailored to the developmental level of the child and take into account pre-existing mental health conditions, temperamental impulsivity.
- Social media may have unique effects on (historically, persistently, or systemically marginalized) or marginalized youth, including exposure to bullying and discrimination but also provides a way to connect with peers, when inaccessible in person.
- Parental/caregiver media literacy and engagement with SM affects youth engagement via modeling and potential problematic Internet usage.

INTRODUCTION
Legal Background

A discussion about social media and youth mental health must be understood in the context of pre-existing laws that absolve social media platforms of legal responsibility for the content of posts. This includes potentially harmful social media posts that encourage self-harm, eating disordered behavior, and suicide as well as threats of physical harm, and cyberbullying.

Section 230 of the Communications Decency Act of 1996[1] states that "No provider or user of an interactive computer service shall be treated as the publisher or speaker

[a] Department of Psychiatry and Behavioral Neuroscience, University of Chicago, 5841 South Maryland Avenue, MC 3077, Chicago, IL 60637, USA; [b] Department of Psychiatry, University of Michigan, 1500 East Medical Center Drive, Spc 5000, Ann Arbor, MI 48109, USA
* Corresponding author.
E-mail address: sanam@bsd.uchicago.edu

Pediatr Clin N Am 72 (2025) 305–316
https://doi.org/10.1016/j.pcl.2024.09.005   **pediatric.theclinics.com**

of any information provided by another information content provider." This act was later applied to social media platforms as they were developed, absolving the companies of liability for user posts. Later, the American Civil Liberties Union (ACLU) and the Queer Resources Directory among others legally challenged the Communications Decency Act, but maintained Section 230 to protect online gathering spaces for marginalized people from regulation.

Subsequent amendments to Section 230 have created exceptions to social media platforms' freedom from liability. The FOSTA-SESTA amendment[1] holds platforms liable for posts or advertisements that facilitated sex trafficking. The "EARN IT" Act of 2020[2] created a commission to "prevent, reduce and respond to the online sexual exploitation of children..." The "SAFE TECH" Act[3] of 2021 removes immunity for social media posts leading to discrimination on the basis of race, sex, religion, and other protected categories. However, this act has been shown to backfire on historically, persistently, or systemically marginalized (HPSM) groups when broad categories of posts are filtered out to avoid lawsuits.

These laws interface with social media companies' restrictions of use by children and adolescents, although they bear no legal responsibility to verify the age of users. Location-based dating apps usually restrict use to age 18 years and older, but Section 230 frees these sites from legal responsibility to ensure users are actually adults. Lesbian, Gay, Bisexual, Transgender, Queer (LGBTQ) + teens lacking opportunities for in-person romantic relationships that heterosexual teens enjoy are likely to go online for these opportunities.[4] Many dating sites fail to require users to report sex offender status, potentially enabling adults to perpetrate sexual abuse upon teens via these apps.

In response to concern from the public about harmful content and abuse of youth on social media platforms, companies have employed content moderation through their community guidelines. These are established set of policies delineating what types of posts will be taken down and the grounds for account suspension. Much can be learned from the history of censorship in entertainment media to ensure the same mistakes are not repeated. The history of entertainment media demonstrates that whether media was censored or not has repeatedly harmed HPSM groups. In 1915, the National Board of Censorship approved Birth of a Nation, a propaganda film for racist ideology, for a general audience. The lack of censorship there spread hate and racism. In 1930, The Motion Picture Production Code delineating 12 categories of censorable "repellent subjects" fit for censorship, including interracial and LGBTQ+ relationships. In this case, the presence of censorship spread hate and racism. Social media companies must learn from the history of censorship in entertainment media lest they repeat it.

Biases Against Historically, Persistently, or Systemically Marginalized Youth

Social media platforms must moderate content in order to protect youth who use them, but some content moderation may unfairly disadvantage members of HPSM groups. A 2021 mixed-methods study[5] found 3 distinct groups of social media users who experienced content and account removals most often: politically conservative participants (whose content was correctly removed because it violated the platforms community guidelines as offensive, misinformation, and adult or hate speech), transgender participants (whose content was removed for being "adult" despite following community guidelines, critical of a dominant group, or specifically related to transgender or queer issues), and Black participants (whose content was incorrectly removed because the post concerned racial justice or racism). They noted that some content is removed despite it not actually violating the community guidelines.

Authors conclude that marginalized social media users are more likely to experience content moderation "false positive and gray areas" and "conservative content removals in the dataset were more likely to represent true positives: content that violated site policies, and thus was correctly removed." This study suggests a lack of consistency and transparency in social media platforms content moderation. Users often report content because it violates their personal norms, which may be prejudiced. Therefore, the process by which content is flagged for removal can privilege majority identities and experiences and further exacerbate systemic inequities.

Automated moderation also has major pitfalls that also are rooted in prejudice. For example, automation of moderation leads to misclassifying African American Vernacular English as hate speech.[5] Automated moderation also removes antiracist posts that are mistakenly being classified as racist.[5] Details of content moderation are vitally important, especially now as Instagram recently announced options to decrease the amount of "sensitive" content that appears in feeds,[6] failing to describe what criteria will be used to label content as "sensitive" content.

There are other ways in which the functioning of social media platforms disadvantage HPSM users. For people who earn their income from content creation on social media, making content less visible without necessarily taking it down may have major economic implications. Sometimes, this phenomenon is referred to as "shadowbanning"—when content is not removed from a platform, but it is strategically hidden instead. There are also reports of replication of an imaginative post created by an HPSM individual by a non-HPSM user whose post becomes more popular. Any underlying prejudices inherent to the inner workings of the social media sites should be rectified. In a society where these prejudices and hatred exist offline, social media sites should make it a priority to eliminate the hate and prejudice in the inner workings of their sites.

Prevalence of Social Media Use

Social media use, pervasive among young people in the United States, has a profound influence in shaping youth culture, communication, and behavior.[7] A recent study conducted by the Pew Research Center[8] highlights the ubiquity of social media use among American adolescents. Nearly all surveyed teens reported having access to a smartphone or a computer, and the majority to a gaming console or tablet, with children in middle and higher income households likely to have access to a home computer.[9] The percentage of adolescents who endorse being online "almost constantly" doubled since the same question was posed a decade earlier. Social media platforms and related use patterns are rapidly evolving, with the most popular platforms for youth as of 2022 to include YouTube, TikTok, Instagram, and Snapchat.[10] Though social media platforms require users to be at least 13 years old, nearly 40% of children between the ages of 8 to 12 years report using social media.[9]

Trends in social media usage vary among subgroups in the United States, including gender and race/ethnicity. Adolescent girls are more likely than teen boys to use TikTok "almost constantly." Boys are more likely to use Discord and Twitch. Black and Hispanic teens are more likely than White teens to be online "almost constantly." Hispanic teens were the most likely to report being on TikTok "almost constantly," though Black teens as a group were most likely to report using TikTok compared to their non-Black peers. White adolescents are more likely to use BeReal but less likely to use all other social media platforms.[11] Indigenous and Asian American Native Hawaiian Pacific Islander youth were not included in the Pew study sample. A survey of adults found that Asian Americans endorse a higher frequency of social media usage than any other racial group.[12]

During the coronavirus disease 2019 (COVID-19) pandemic, social distancing practices and school closures limited the ability of children and adolescents to socialize in person, contributing to the rapid escalation in their social media use. Between 2019 and 2021, the average amount of daily screen media exposure increased by nearly an hour among tweens, and well over an hour among teens.[9] Among US children aged 8 to 12 years, screen time increased by 1.75 hours daily during the early pandemic and later remained above prepandemic levels by 1.11 hours. This study found screen time was higher among children of Black race or Hispanic ethnicity, older children, and children whose mothers lacked a college education.[13] A cross-sectional study found that 12 to 13 year old children were using social media an average of 0.98 hours per day.[14] Social media platforms afforded the opportunity for one-to-one communication, mutual online friendships, as well as positive online experiences, which mitigated feelings of loneliness and stress during COVID-19-related social distancing.[15] More than ever, social media is part of the everyday life of American youth with consequences for their mental health.

Social Media Effects on Mental Health

Social media shapes the ways youth understand themselves, the world around them, and how they fit into it. Social media can both benefit and harm the mental health of youth.[16–18] Social media's contribution to both ill-being and well-being occurs on separate spectrums.[19] For example, watching videos on YouTube for hours may evoke positive emotions and contribute to well-being, while simultaneously displacing quality time with family and friends, creating loneliness and ill-being. Similarly, social media use may make equal contributions to both well-being and ill-being. See **Fig. 1**A–C for additional examples. Social media often disrupts sleep and displaces physical activity and in-person interactions, all of which are critical for healthy development and emotion regulation.[20] Social media can exacerbate experiences of bullying and discrimination, increasing risk for negative mental health outcomes including anxiety, depression, and trauma-related symptoms.[21] Involvement with cyberbullying is also associated with an increased risk of suicidal behavior and suicide attempt.[22,23] Exposure to highly curated social media posts depicting idealized version of a peer's physical appearance, life events, or social engagements invites unrealistic comparisons that can adversely affect self-image and elevate risks for mental health concerns including anxiety, depression, and eating disorders.[24]

In a recent 2023 study, participants aged 16 to 21 years in Norway completed online questionnaires about their social media use and mental health.[25] Exploratory factor

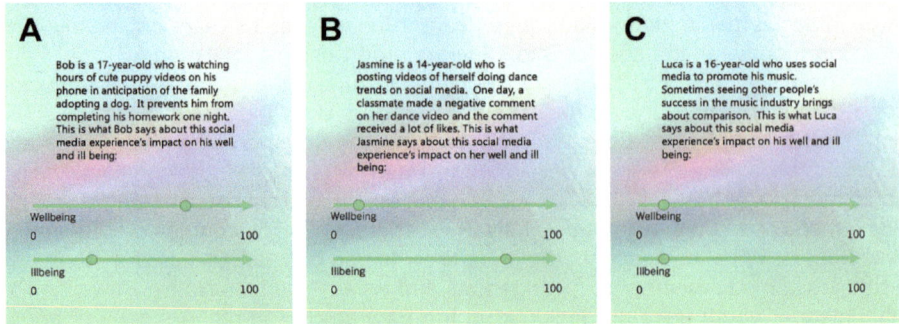

Fig. 1. (*A–C*) Mini case vignettes: social media experiences lead to unique impacts on well-being and ill-being for different individuals.

analysis found 3 main factors correlated with negative mental health: subjective social media overuse (included feeling "addicted"), social obligations (included fearing missing out or failing obligations to comment on friends' posts), and source of concern (included feeling overwhelmed on social media and worries that use is unhealthy or is being monitored). Of these 3 factors, the factor "source of concern" had the largest association with mental health problems and the weakest association with self-reported amount of time spent on social media. Reaction to any given experience on social media (eg, viewing post about a news story on Instagram) vary significantly depending on characteristics of the user. Users high in "source of concern" may notice that social media is making them feel overwhelmed or monitored and respond by using social media less often or employ certain tactics to minimize harm. Social media platforms do provide unique opportunities for peer engagement, eliciting emotional support or community, and creative outlets that may contribute significantly to well-being.

Effects Specific to Historically, Persistently, or Systemically Marginalized Youth

Social media engagement confers risks and benefits that are universal to all teens, though some factors are specific to HPSM youth. Research documenting the relationship between social media and mental health of youth is relatively new and incomplete, particularly data regarding its unique impacts on youth from HPSM communities. Few studies focus on social media influences on marginalized racial, ethnic, sexual, gender, socioeconomic backgrounds, or differently abled youth.[26] For youth who lack access to peers with shared identities, experiences, or interests in their local communities, social media may facilitate valuable connection with these otherwise inaccessible individuals. Studies of HPSM youth demonstrate that social media can provide social support, identity affirmation and development, and community, allowing youth to feel more accepted.[27] Lesbian, Gay, Bisexual, Transgender, Queer, Intersex, Asexual + (other identities) (LGBTQIA+) youth reticent to inquire about related health information or disclose their identities with caregivers or local peers may benefit by doing so via social media.[28] LGBTQIA+ youth use social media to seek information about LGBTQIA+-related health, news, and representation, as well as obtain emotional support, and explore aspects of their identity.[29]

However, while social media may be protective for members of marginalized groups in some ways, it may also confer uniquely elevated risk for harm. For example, social media-based bullying, which disproportionately affects female adolescents and sexual minority youth, is consistently associated with the risk of depression.[30,31] LGBTQIA+ and female adolescents are more likely to experience online harassment and abuse, and suffer associated emotional consequences, including sadness, anxiety, and worry. Several studies demonstrate links between social media use and mental health problems (poor sleep related to social media use, depressive symptoms, poor body image, and eating disorders) find a greater association for girls.[32–34] Multiple experimental studies show that viewing idealized and filtered images on social media worsened body dissatisfaction and have been linked to disordered eating, depressive symptoms, and low self-esteem, particularly among adolescent girls.[35,36]

Youth of color face specific risks and benefits with regard to their social media engagement, which are mediated by cultural factors and mental health vulnerabilities. They may benefit from racial-ethnic social norms informing identity but often encounter stereotyping, racism, and even traumatic experiences. Exposure to individual and vicarious social media racial discrimination has been found to exacerbate depressive symptoms and substance use problems.[37] Another study found adolescents exposed to online hate messaging are more likely to suffer depression and social anxiety. In this study, the association between social media use frequency and depressive symptoms was stronger in Asian Americans, while the association between social media use and social anxiety was reversed among Black youth.[38] Viewing of race-related traumatic events (eg, videos of race-based violence) has been linked to symptoms of posttraumatic stress disorder and depression, particularly for those who are Latinx or female individuals.[21] Black youth utilize social media to obtain social support regarding race-based traumatic events online, which may mitigate related psychological distress.[21] Adolescents of color experience online racial discrimination at high rates and suffer associated depression, anxiety, and trauma-related symptoms.[39]

Youth with intersectional identities may be subject to compounded stressors related to their multiple identities. One-third adolescent girls of color report exposure to racist content or language on social media platforms at least monthly.[40] Some encounter social media "beauty filters," which apply skin tones or facial features that are typically associated with White people, further contributing to racially biased beauty standards. Stereotyped depictions of youth with marginalized identities pose culturally specific risks of discrimination and negative self-image.[41] A recent study demonstrated that social media usage among Black and Asian American adolescent girls was associated with increased emphasis on sexual appeal and physical appearance compared to White girls, possibly related to shame caused by such racially biased body ideals and stereotypes as well as fetishization.[24]

Social Media Modulation

A 2022 study found that many youth employ strategies to moderate their social media use.[42] Over 800 participants aged 14 to 24 years responded to questions about advice they would give to someone who is new to social media, if they had ever felt the need to change something about their social media use and if they had ever deleted or thought about deleting a social media account. They expressed concern about the amount of time spent on social media and sometimes experienced challenges in cutting down their use. They also expressed concern about the content they consumed on social media, including edited photos and misinformation. They also worried about what they posted both in terms of their own safety and their interpersonal interactions with others on social media. Many employed settings or features of the app itself to moderate their use, and most reported thinking about deleting a social media account or app or actually doing so. Some described how they changed their social media use for the sake of wellness.

- "I had to manually block content I felt was negatively affecting me and force myself to take time away from certain apps"
- "I realized that I was only following celebrities and seeing their heavily edited photos and taking them in as reality. When I ended that, I was following only meme accounts and was wasting hours and hours on them so I narrowed my account to only my friends"
- "I kind of regret how easy I've made it to find out things about me online so I've considered deleting some accounts and starting over to blur my efootprint a bit"
- "I set reminders on when to get off"
- "I have an iPhone and it shows me how much time I spend on social media"
- "I was sending too much time on TikTok, and it was messing with my head so I told myself that I will not go on it last like 9 PM."

Many youth understand how best to moderate their social media use, and providers can help to disseminate these tips and tricks to their peers who struggle. Another study indicated that social media users' ability to employ sophisticated techniques to regulate their use depended largely on their knowledge of technology.[43] An individual's knowledge about such techniques seems likely to depend also on having received related formal education, their peer group, conversations with caregivers, and their own curiosity among other factors. All youth should be educated on how social media can affect their well-being, overall media literacy, techniques to moderate use, and digital citizenship.

Formal school-based education on these topics would be invaluable for students. A number of social media education programs have been tested in the school setting,[44] and some states introduced legislation, which would add such education to school curriculums.[45] Social media education can also occur in the doctor's office. This may require that providers learn about healthy social media modification techniques themselves. A 2022 study found that a video designed to improve provider knowledge and comfortability with giving guidance about implementing changes on Instagram via the in-app settings showed promise.[46] Provider understanding about hiding "like" and "view" counts on Instagram showed the greatest gains. After watching this video, providers could better enable young patients to make social media setting changes, and this could even happen during a clinical visit.

It is also important for social media companies to partner with mental health professionals in the ongoing development of setting modifications so healthy changes are available and beneficial. Meta issued an announcement in early 2024 that Facebook and Instagram will hide potentially harmful content for users aged under 18 years.[6] Now youth searching for content related to suicide, self-harm, or eating disorders on these platforms will be redirected to help resources. However, youth tend to use unrelated hashtags to prevent their posts from being taken down by social media apps due to community violations.[47] Social media platforms set community guidelines[48–50] for what types of content will be taken down by the platform (eg, graphic violent/sexual content, threats, or the sale of regulated goods). However, there is some content that may not violate their guidelines but is still sensitive in some way. Instagram now has opportunities for users to control the amount of sensitive content they are presented with. They also have an option to allow for increased "fact checking," which moves content that is "false, partly false, altered or content with missing context" to lower in the person's feed. As mentioned in the history section earlier, there is a need for platform transparency related to how facts are checked and the sensitive nature of content is determined. Social media sites must use caution so that misclassifications of content do not propagate bias, racism, and hate.

Role of Parents and Caregivers

Parents/caregivers play a critical role in navigating the impact of social media on children and adolescents. Caregivers who are involved in regulating their children's media consumption and enjoy greater digital literacy may be best positioned to protect them against unhealthy social media habits and experiences. Caregiver mediation refers to parents/caregivers' management of the time youth spend using media, as well as restrictions on and explanations about content, in order to mitigate harm and maximize benefit.[51] Caregiver mediation may involve ongoing discussions about social media experiences, restricting content inappropriate for a child's level of maturity, and establishing clear rules for social media use. Caregivers who are active social media users themselves may benefit from greater digital literacy about social media content and influencers and enjoy a clearer perspective on their children's engagement.[52] A number of related studies indicate parental/caregiver mediation may boost adolescents' well-being and protect against ill-being.[53]

A caregiver's own engagement with social media greatly affects the impact of media on their children. Several studies indicate that children's media engagement reflects their caregiver's use.[54,55] Another demonstrated that adolescents with moderate-to-severe problematic Internet use (PIU) were almost 3 times as likely to have caregivers with PIU themselves. Excessive caregiver social media use can displace essential parent/caregiver–child interactions, which may result in children seeking care and attention in unhealthy ways, including excessive social media use. Caregiver social media posts about their children (ie, "sharenting") are common and may risk violating children's digital autonomy and confidentiality. Less common are caregivers who rely on family-based social media posts for income, presenting additional complications for the well-being and development of their children.[56,57]

Given children's progressive engagement with social media and the growing recognition of how that engagement may affect their health and development, the American Academy of Pediatrics and the American Academy of Child and Adolescent Psychiatry recommend the establishment of a family media plan and provide specific guidance on social media. Parents and caregivers are advised to identify what content they are exposed to on social media, to determine if that content is developmentally appropriate, a source of vicarious prejudice, or includes bullying or abuse. Caregivers should consider limiting access to devices and restricting age-inappropriate materials via device-specific and platform-specific parental controls. Parents/caregivers must consider the effects of their own media habits in family media planning.

CLINICS CARE POINTS

- Social media use has unique contributions to both ill-being and well-being.
- Recommendations about social media use should be tailored to the developmental level of the child and take into account pre-existing mental health conditions, temperamental impulsivity, and history with bullying.
- Recommend that caregivers develop a family media plan regarding use of media devices, including social media.
- Educate youth and families about potentially harmful content and identifying misinformation.
- Assess how patients use social media and to what extent.
- Ask parents/caregivers how they model social media use, including if/how they share information about their children.
- Inquire about exposure to cyberbullying, discrimination, and racism.
- Discuss how viewing highly curated and idealized online images can impact self-esteem.
- Advise caregivers to limit exposure to content that encourages self-harm, eating disordered behavior, suicide, stereotypes, or prejudice.
- Support HPSM youth and their families in a culturally sensitive manner.
- Identify problematic social media use, which displaces in-person relationships, sleep, physical activity, academics, and so forth.
- Recognize how social media affects risks for depression, anxiety, trauma-related symptoms, and eating disorders.
- Social media may offer unique benefits for individuals who are uncomfortable expressing LGBTQIA+ identities in person or feel unwelcome by or disconnected to their local communities.
- Consider helping patients to make healthy changes to social media settings.

Resources

- American Academy of Child and Adolescent Psychiatry (AACAP) Policy Statement on the Impact of Social Media on Youth Mental Health https://www.aacap.org/AACAP/Policy_Statements/2023/Social_Media_Youth_Mental_Health.aspx

- American Academy of Child and Adolescent Psychiatry Facts for Families on Social Media and Teens https://www.aacap.org/AACAP/Families_and_Youth/Facts_for_Families/FFF-Guide/Social-Media-and-Teens-100.aspx

- American Psychological Association Health Advisory on Social Media Use in Adolescence https://www.apa.org/topics/social-media-internet/health-advisory-adolescent-social-media-use.pdf

- The U.S. Surgeon General's Advisory: Social Media and Youth Mental Health https://www.hhs.gov/sites/default/files/sg-youth-mental-health-social-media-advisory.pdf

- American Academy of Pediatrics Family Media Plan https://www.healthychildren.org/English/fmp/Pages/MediaPlan.aspx

- American Academy of Pediatrics Center of Excellence on Social Media and Youth Mental Health https://www.aap.org/en/patient-care/media-and-children/center-of-excellence-on-social-media-and-youth-mental-health/#: ~ :text=What%20We%20Do,protect%20youth%20mental%20health%20online

- Research-based tips from pediatricians for families (AAP) https://downloads.aap.org/AAP/PDF/CoE_one_pager_with_disclaimer.pdf

---

DISCLOSURE

J. Harness has received research support from AFSP Young Investigator Award, Ouida Scholar Award (Michigan Medicine), and Research Scouts Award (Michigan Medicine). S. Anam is partially supported by grants from Substance Abuse and Mental Health Services Administration (SAMHSA) (1 H79 SM087864-01) and National Institutes of Health (NIH) (NIH 1RO1MH132792-01). She has received research support from University of Chicago Provost's Global Faculty Awards and the Dean's Fund for Faculty Research.

REFERENCES

1. Section 230: an overview. 2024. Available at: https://crsreports.congress.gov/product/pdf/R/R46751#: ~ :text=%E2%80%94No%20provider%20or%20user%20of,by%20another%20information%20content%20provider. Accessed February 6, 2024.
2. S.3398 - EARN IT Act of 2020. Congress.gov; 2020. Available at: https://www.congress.gov/bill/116th-congress/senate-bill/3398/text. Accessed February 6, 2024.
3. H.R.3421 - SAFE TECH Act. Congress.gov; 2021. Available at: https://www.congress.gov/bill/117th-congress/house-bill/3421?q=%7B%22search%22%3A%22Safeguarding+Against+Fraud%2C+Exploitation%2C+Threats%2C+Extremism+and+Consumer+Harms+Act+of+2021%22%7D&s=1&r=7&s=1&r=11. Accessed February 6, 2024.
4. Suto DJ, Macapagal K, Turban JL. Geosocial networking application use among sexual minority adolescents. J Am Acade Child Adolesc Psychiatry 2021;60(4):429–31.
5. Haimson OL, Delmonaco D, Nie P, et al. Disproportionate removals and differing content moderation experiences for conservative, transgender, and Black social

media users: marginalization and moderation gray areas. Proc ACM Hum-Comput Interact 2021;5(CSCW2):1–35.

6. Dara Kerr. Under growing pressure, Meta vows to make it harder for teens to see harmful content. npr. Published January 23, 2024. Available at: https://www.npr.org/2024/01/09/1223583540/meta-harmful-content-instagram-harder-teens-facebook. Accessed January 23, 2024.

7. Social media and youth mental health, the U.S. Surgeon General's advisory. 2023. Available at: https://www.hhs.gov/sites/default/files/sg-youth-mental-health-social-media-advisory.pdf.

8. Emily A. Vogels AND RISA GELLES-WATNICK. Teens and social media: Key Findings from Pew research Center surveys. Pew research Center; 2023. Available at: https://www.pewresearch.org/short-reads/2023/04/24/teens-and-social-media-key-findings-from-pew-research-center-surveys/. Accessed January 31, 2024.

9. Rideout V, Robb M. The role of media during the pandemic: connection, Creativity, and learning for tweens and teens. Common Sense media; 2021. Available at: https://www.commonsensemedia.org/sites/default/files/research/report/8-18-role-of-media-research-report-final-web.pdf. Accessed February 1, 2024.

10. Emily A. Vogels, Risa Gelles-Watnick and Navid Massarat. Teens, social media and technology 2022. Pew research Center; 2022. Available at: file:///Users/janeehar/Downloads/PI_2022.08.10_Teens-and-Tech_FINAL.pdf. Accessed September 25, 2022.

11. Anderson M, Faverio M, Gottfried J. Teens, social media and Technology 2023. Pew Research Center; 2023. Available at: https://www.pewresearch.org/internet/2023/12/11/teens-social-media-and-technology-2023/.

12. Charmaraman L, Chan HB, Chen S, et al. Asian American social media use: from cyber dependence and cyber harassment to saving face. Asian Am J Psychol 2018;9(1):72–86.

13. Hedderson MM, Bekelman TA, Li M, et al. Trends in screen time use among children during the COVID-19 pandemic, july 2019 through August 2021. JAMA Netw Open 2023;6(2):e2256157.

14. Nagata JM, Abdel Magid HS, Pettee Gabriel K. Screen time for children and adolescents during the coronavirus disease 2019 pandemic. Obesity 2020;28(9):1582–3.

15. Marciano L, Ostroumova M, Schulz PJ, et al. Digital media use and adolescents' mental health during the Covid-19 pandemic: a systematic review and meta-analysis. Front Public Health 2022;9:793868.

16. Khalaf AM, Alubied AA, Khalaf AM, et al. The impact of social media on the mental health of adolescents and young adults: a systematic review. Cureus 2023. https://doi.org/10.7759/cureus.42990.

17. Moreno MA, Radesky J. Putting forward a new narrative for adolescent media: the American Academy of Pediatrics Center of Excellence on social media and youth mental health. J Adolesc Health 2023;73(2):227–9.

18. Santos RMS, Mendes CG, Sen Bressani GY, et al. The associations between screen time and mental health in adolescents: a systematic review. BMC Psychol 2023;11(1):127.

19. Valkenburg PM, Meier A, Beyens I. Social media use and its impact on adolescent mental health: an umbrella review of the evidence. Curr Opin Psychol 2022;44:58–68.

20. Chalermchutidej W, Manaboriboon B, Sanpawitayakul G, et al. Sleep, social media use and mental health in female adolescents aged 12 to 18 years old during the COVID-19 pandemic. BMC Pediatr 2023;23(1):398.
21. Tynes BM, Willis HA, Stewart AM, et al. Race-related traumatic events online and mental health among adolescents of color. J Adolesc Health 2019;65(3):371–7.
22. Nixon C. Current perspectives: the impact of cyberbullying on adolescent health. AHMT 2014;143. https://doi.org/10.2147/AHMT.S36456.
23. John A, Glendenning AC, Marchant A, et al. Self-harm, suicidal behaviours, and cyberbullying in children and young people: systematic review. J Med Internet Res 2018;20(4):e129.
24. Ward LM, Jerald MC, Grower P, et al. Primping, performing, and policing: social media use and self-sexualization among U.S. White, Black, and Asian-American adolescent girls. Body Image 2023;46:324–35.
25. Finserås T, Hjetland G, Sivertsen B, et al. Reexploring problematic social media use and its relationship with adolescent mental health. Findings from the "LifeOnSoMe"-study. PRBM 2023;16:5101–11.
26. American Psychological Association. Health Advisory on Social Media Use in Adolescents. 2023. Available at: https://www.apa.org/topics/social-media-internet/health-advisory-adolescent-social-media-use. (Accessed 31 January 2024).
27. Karim S, Choukas-Bradley S, Radovic A, et al. Support over social media among socially Isolated sexual and gender minority youth in Rural U.S. During the COVID-19 pandemic: opportunities for Intervention research. Int J Environ Res Public Health 2022;19(23):15611.
28. Craig SL, Eaton AD, McInroy LB, et al. Can social media participation enhance LGBTQ+ youth well-being? Development of the social media benefits Scale. Social Media + Society 2021;7(1):2056305112198893.
29. Paceley MS. Gender and sexual minority youth in nonmetropolitan communities: individual- and community-level needs for support. Fam Soc 2016;97(2):77–85.
30. Alhajji M, Bass S, Dai T. Cyberbullying, mental health, and violence in adolescents and associations with sex and race: data from the 2015 youth risk behavior survey. Global Pediatric Health 2019;6. 2333794X1986888.
31. Hamm MP, Newton AS, Chisholm A, et al. Prevalence and effect of cyberbullying on children and young people: a scoping review of social media studies. JAMA Pediatr 2015;169(8):770.
32. Kelly Y, Zilanawala A, Booker C, et al. Social media use and adolescent mental health: findings from the UK millennium cohort study. EClinicalMedicine 2018;6:59–68.
33. Alonzo R, Hussain J, Stranges S, et al. Interplay between social media use, sleep quality, and mental health in youth: a systematic review. Sleep Med Rev 2021;56:101414.
34. Twenge JM, Haidt J, Lozano J, et al. Specification curve analysis shows that social media use is linked to poor mental health, especially among girls. Acta Psychol 2022;224:103512.
35. Thai H, Davis CG, Mahboob W, et al. Reducing social media use improves appearance and weight esteem in youth with emotional distress. Psychology of Popular Media 2024;13(1):162–9.
36. Mabe AG, Forney KJ, Keel PK. Do you "like" my photo? Facebook use maintains eating disorder risk: Facebook Use Maintains Risk. Int J Eat Disord 2014;47(5):516–23.
37. Tao X, Fisher CB. Exposure to social media racial discrimination and mental health among adolescents of color. J Youth Adolescence 2022;51(1):30–44.

38. Hernandez JM, Charmaraman L, Schaefer HS. Conceptualizing the role of racial–ethnic identity in U.S. adolescent social technology use and well-being. Transl Issues Psychol Sci 2023;9(3):199–215.

39. Galán CA, Tung I, Tabachnick AR, et al. Combating the conspiracy of silence: clinician recommendations for talking about racism-related events with youth of color. J Am Acade Child Adolesc Psychiatry 2022;61(5):586–90.

40. Nesi J, Mann S, Robb MB. (2023). Teens and mental health: how girls really feel about social media. San Francisco, CA: Common Sense. Available at: https://www.jaacap.org/article/S0890-8567(23)00079-5/fulltext. (Accessed 31 January 2024).

41. Pak TK, Kiriella DA, Adiba A, et al. Shang-chi and the legend of the ten rings. directed by destin daniel cretton. marvel studios; 2021. J Am Acade Child Adolesc Psychiatry 2023;62(6):700–1.

42. Harness J, Fitzgerald K, Sullivan H, et al. Youth Insight about social media effects on well/ill-being and self-modulating efforts. J Adolesc Health 2022;71(3):324–33.

43. Nguyen MH. Managing social media use in an "always-on" society: EXPLORING digital wellbeing strategies that people use to disconnect. Mass Commun Soc 2021;24(6):795–817.

44. Domoff S, Borgen A, Rye B, et al. Problematic digital media use and addiction. In: Nesi J, Telzer E, Prinstein M, editors. Handbook of adolescent digital media use and mental health. Cambridge: Cambridge University Press; 2022. p. 300–16.

45. SENATE. No. 588 State of New Jersey 220th Legislature. 2022. Available at: https://pub.njleg.state.nj.us/Bills/2022/S1000/588_I1.PDF. Accessed February 6, 2024.

46. Harness J, Mohiuddin S. Advising modulation of social media use with patients: how an educational video for medical trainees shows promise. Acad Psychiatry 2022. https://doi.org/10.1007/s40596-022-01736-8.

47. Moreno MA, Ton A, Selkie E, et al. Secret society 123: understanding the language of self-harm on Instagram. J Adolesc Health 2016;58(1):78–84.

48. Community guidelines. Available at: https://www.youtube.com/howyoutubeworks/policies/community-guidelines/. Accessed February 6, 2024.

49. Community guidelines. Available at: https://help.instagram.com/477434105621119. Accessed February 6, 2024.

50. Community guidelines. Available at: https://www.tiktok.com/community-guidelines/en/. Accessed February 6, 2024.

51. Beyens I, Keijsers L, Coyne SM. Social media, parenting, and well-being. Current Opinion Psychol 2022;47:101350.

52. Lin MH, Vijayalakshmi A, Laczniak R. Toward an understanding of parental views and actions on social media influencers targeted at adolescents: the roles of parents' social media use and empowerment. Front Psychol 2019;10:2664.

53. Cohen A, Bendelow A, Smith T, et al. Parental attitudes on social media monitoring for youth: cross-sectional survey study. JMIR Pediatr Parent 2023;6:e46365.

54. Geurts SM, Koning IM, Vossen HGM, et al. Rules, role models or overall climate at home? Relative associations of different family aspects with adolescents' problematic social media use. Compr Psychiatry 2022;116:152318.

55. Lauricella AR, Cingel DP. Parental influence on youth media use. J Child Fam Stud 2020;29(7):1927–37.

56. Garrido F, Alvarez A, González-Caballero JL, et al. Description of the exposure of the most-followed spanish instamoms' children to social media. Int J Environ Res Public Health 2023;20(3):2426.

57. Jorge A, Marôpo L, Coelho AM, et al. Mummy influencers and professional sharenting. Eur J Cult Stud 2022;25(1):166–82.

Youth Digital Dilemmas

Exploring the Intersection Between Social Media and Anxiety

Merlin Ariefdjohan, PhD, MPH[a,1], Dana Reid, DO[b,1],
Sandra Fritsch, MD, MSEd, DFAACAP[a,c,*]

KEYWORDS

- Social media • Youth • Anxiety • Screen habits

KEY POINTS

- The prevalence of anxiety disorders, already the most common behavioral health conditions in youth and teens, is increasing over the last decade. Social media and other screen habits and experiences impact the development of youth and may promote or worsen disorders of anxiety.
- Given the potential effects of increased exposure to social media, "healthy" digital habits are essential to mitigate harm.
- Elevated exposure to social media has given rise to new manifestations of anxiety among youth (eg, nomophobia, fear of missing out, cyberchondria, among others).
- Social media can benefit youth via transmission of knowledge and facilitating peer support.
- Understanding the connections between use of social media and anxiety is an evolving area of study. Current literature has focused on studies that include anxiety as a variable alongside other indicators of mental health, such as depression, suicidality, loneliness, and others. Providers must stay abreast of this evolving field of study.

INTRODUCTION

Most of the world's population, including youth, regularly access the digital world for learning, recreation, commerce, working, and/or socializing. In October 2023, an estimated 5.3 billion of the worldwide population of 8.1 billion used social media.[1] Over the last twenty years, social media engagement has surged dramatically, growing

[a] Department of Psychiatry, University of Colorado Anschutz Medical Campus, Aurora, CO 80045, USA; [b] Private Practice, Alpharetta, GA 30022, USA; [c] Pediatric Mental Health Institute, Children's Hospital Colorado, Aurora, CO 80045, USA
[1] Denotes co-first authorship to recognize equally significant contribution.
* Corresponding author. Pediatric Mental Health Institute, Children's Hospital Colorado, 13123 East 16th Avenue, Mailstop: B130, Aurora, CO 80045.
E-mail address: Sandra.fritsch@childrenscolorado.org

Pediatr Clin N Am 72 (2025) 317–331
https://doi.org/10.1016/j.pcl.2024.09.006
pediatric.theclinics.com
0031-3955/25/© 2024 Elsevier Inc. All rights reserved, including those for text and data mining, AI training, and similar technologies.

from 5% in the United States in 2005 to nearly 70% worldwide today.[1,2] Merriam-Webster defines social media as "forms of electronic communication (such as websites for social networking and microblogging) through which users create online communities to share information, ideas, personal messages, and other content (such as videos)."[3] In December 2023, the Pew Research Center released findings from an online survey of 1453 US teens, indicating that YouTube, TikTok, Snapchat, and Instagram are the online platforms used most by American adolescents.[4]

Access and the use of handheld screen devices (eg, smartphones) has increased in youth of all ages. In 2017, nearly 95% of all children (0–8 years) in the United States had exposure and/or individual access to a smartphone, up from the 63% reported in 2013.[5] The Pew survey indicated that 95% of US teens aged 13 to 17 years own a smartphone.[4] Survey results indicated that 50% of older teens were constant Internet users, as compared to 40% of younger teens.[4] The increased use of smartphones and other screen devices has been accompanied by elevated exposure to social media.[5] Alarmingly, nearly 40% of youth aged 8 to 12 years use social media despite the standard age requirement for social media being set at 13 years.[6] Further, socializing in a distant, asynchronous manner via social media may be appealing for youth suffering anxiety disorders, as it allows for avoidance of anxiety-producing situations including the immediacy of potentially awkward in-person social interactions and the need to leave the home environment.

Anxiety is the most common mental health condition among youth, with a lifetime prevalence reported at 28.8% and a median age of onset noted at 11 years.[7] The presentation of anxiety in children and teens changes developmentally, with separation anxiety disorder presenting in younger children and increasing through midchildhood, social anxiety disorder generally manifesting in early adolescence, and generalized anxiety disorder typically emerging in later adolescence and early adulthood.[8] The prevalence of anxiety among youth increased by nearly 30% from 2016 to 2019, predating the COVID-19 pandemic.[9] Soaring rates of pediatric mental illness following the COVID-19 pandemic led to a declaration of a pediatric mental health national emergency by the American Academy of Pediatrics (AAP) in 2021, followed by the US Surgeon General's advisory "Protecting Youth Mental Health" which includes 20 references to social media.[10,11]

The rise in mental health needs and anxiety among young individuals mirror increases in screen time and social media usage in the same population, suggesting a significant relationship. A research study with 17,409 youth in the United Kingdom found that the impact of social media on life satisfaction varied during specific age ranges in adolescence. For male individuals, the critical periods were at ages 14 to 15 years and 19 years, while for females, it was at ages 11 to 13 years and 19 years. The study further showed that higher social media use predicted lower life satisfaction 1 year later, and vice versa, depending on these age groups.[12] A recent longitudinal cohort study of kindergarteners in Shanghai, China, sought to understand the relationship of screen time, screen content, and mental health.[13] Exposure to educational screen media was not found to be a risk factor for mental health difficulties, but both screen time and social media exposure were.[13] While causation is yet to be proven, findings from multiple correlational studies have sparked major concerns about the influence of social media on the mental health of young individuals. This has led to the issuance of an advisory issued in 2023 by the US Surgeon General warning that social media use may adversely affect youth mental health.[14]

Research exploring the impact of social media on mental health is rapidly evolving, as is related policy development. This article serves as a brief review of the current literature on the interplay of social media and anxiety among youth living in the digital age. It discusses potential risks and benefits of social media use for youth and offers strategies for preventing and managing social media-induced anxiety.

A BRIEF REVIEW OF THE LITERATURE

While causation remains unproven, research suggests an association between excessive social media exposure and elevated anxiety.[15–17] A longitudinal study on a community sample of teens living in Canada (aged 13–14 years at the initial time of the study, and then followed up a year later) evaluated how social media use (ie, passive, active, and problematic) predicts depression and anxiety symptoms.[18] Active and problematic social media use was associated with subsequent anxiety symptoms, with extraversion moderating these effects.[18]

Exposure to social media has been associated with heightened anxiety for a variety of reasons. Youth with active social media engagement may base self-worth on their number of likes and followers, and disappointing social media response may lead to worries about status and self-efficacy. A 3-year longitudinal study of sixth and seventh graders in rural North Carolina, United States, found that habitual social media checking may alter brain sensitivity to social rewards, evidenced by changes in functional MRI.[19] Comparing peers' social media posts may influence self-worth development, and potentially harm self-esteem. Realizing that peers have more followers or likes makes one feel less popular, likable, and interesting, potentially exacerbating low self-esteem and social anxiety.[19]

Social media users curate an online persona by posting the most positive images experiences, achievements, and accomplishments, contributing to a false impression of peers and unfair social comparisons. A survey of Singapore youth found higher levels of engagement in Instagram were positively correlated with social anxiety.[20] Due to this tendency toward positive self-presentation, users who excessively use social media can find themselves struggling with upward social comparisons, mistakenly perceive themselves as inferior.[21] These tendencies can adversely impact self-esteem and trigger social anxiety.[21,22]

The tendency of social media to exacerbate anxiety may disproportionately affect female adolescents. The Quebec Longitudinal Study of Child Development investigated the relationships of generalized and social anxiety with Internet use among Canadian teens.[23] Girls who started using the Internet for social engagements at the age of 15 years had a higher likelihood of having generalized anxiety and social anxiety when they reached 17 years of age. In contrast, no relationship between Internet use and mental health symptoms was found for boys.[23] A longitudinal study on individuals aged 10 to 15 years in the United Kingdom assessed the time spent on social media at ages 12 to 13 years, followed by measuring self-esteem and social connectedness between the ages of 13 and 15 years, and finally evaluating mental health at ages 14 to 15 years.[24] Findings revealed a linear trend linking increased social media time to deteriorating mental health. This trend was potentially moderated by positive self-esteem, although the association was not statistically significant.[24] Further longitudinal research is needed to elucidate the relationship between social media use and anxiety, and how this relationship changes across stages of development and varies by gender.

Adolescents may feel pressured to project idealized online images, which can subsequently cause or exacerbate anxiety. Edited and filtered images and videos posted online create unrealistic standards. Social media algorithms reinforce these expectations by favoring content similar to what teens are already viewing. Adolescents unconsciously internalize the unattainable beauty standards set by social media profiles despite rationally understanding that they may not represent reality. Youth may feel the pressure to compete with idealized peer profiles by using editing apps and filters to alter their facial and body features and post flawless images of themselves. This cycle, particularly affecting girls, can lead to dissatisfaction with appearance, doing excessive photo editing, and an increased vulnerability to anxiety.[23,25] Frequent social media engagement may thus foster unrealistic body ideals and lead to body dysmorphic disorder, eating disorders, anxiety, and depression.[23,26]

Social media also has positive effects. It provides an alternative means for socially anxious youth to practice social skills and connect with others, which can be perceived as being less intimidating than traditional face-to-face interactions. An Italian study explored the impact of social media on highly socially anxious teens compared to peers.[27] This cross-sectional study found that socially anxious teens perceived asynchronicity offered through social media interaction as a positive feature since it allows users to take time to craft a social response.[27] Conversely, social media posts often trigger fears of judgment, leading to rumination and self-doubt. This overthinking can spiral to thoughts such as "did I offend someone?" or "did what I post sound stupid or awkward?" resulting in compulsively checking posts to assess likes and comments or needless re-editing. A study of 1740 college students in China found a positive correlation between passive social media use (ie, looking at other's posts without commenting or posting oneself) and social anxiety, while active use showed a negative correlation.[16] The study suggests that socially anxious teens may improve their communication skills by actively engaging in social media, instead of being passive users.[16] Improved communication skills could enhance self-esteem, resulting in more positive online interactions that might carry over to improving in-person social engagements.

NEW TERMINOLOGY FOR POTENTIAL ASSOCIATION OF SOCIAL MEDIA AND ANXIETY

The evolving and pervasive nature of the digital world, has led to the following terms for contemporary social media-related anxieties.

Nomophobia

Nomophobia, short for "no mobile phone phobia," refers to the fear of being without a smartphone or not being unable to connect to social media. A recent systematic review found nomophobia was endorsed by 15.2% to 99.7% of youth, depending on age, gender, location, and daily usage.[28] An unhealthy overreliance on smartphones to maintain a near-constant social media connection can negatively impact academic performance, sleep quality, and anxiety-inducing habits.[28,29]

Fear of Missing Out

"Fear of missing out" (FOMO) is linked to excessive social media use. Daily exposure to social media to curated photos of peers having fun, looking good, or celebrating achievements can make youth feel excluded, inferior, lonely, and inadequate.[30,31] These feelings are related to a sense of regret for failing to have similar experiences and may result in an intense need for immediate social engagement.[32] Teens experiencing FOMO compulsively monitor social media activities to stay updated, often intensifying the cycle of feeling excluded. Habitual checking habits can be problematic for some youth (eg, by constantly interrupting important tasks or in-person socializing), especially those who may be predisposed to obsessive compulsive disorder. Any combination of social comparison, negative online interactions, and FOMO could elevate stress and anxiety[31,33] that subsequently detract from sleep quality, academic performance, overall mood, and well-being.[18,30,32,34]

Cyberchondria

The Internet has become a massive repository of knowledge, both accurate and inaccurate. Individuals contribute to and extract information at will. Health information circulating on the Internet is largely unregulated and may lack factual verification.[35] Individuals may compulsively search for health information online, misinterpret normal experiences as signs of severe illness, and eschew seeking professional medical advice.[36,37] Increased tendency to conduct self-diagnoses via the Internet has given rise to "cyberchondria", which is defined as an excessive anxiety of having a severe medical condition as triggered by information obtained through online research and social media.[38] With the advent of TikTok, health care providers are seeing youth utilizing social media mental health content to self-diagnose mental health conditions.[39] A recent meta-analysis noted a significant positive correlation between seeking health information online and anxiety, and between anxiety and cyberchondria.[37] Seeking information through copious Internet searches can also lead to information overload and decision fatigue, which may further elicit greater anxiety, and consequently creating a vicious cycle.[40]

STRATEGIES FOR MANAGING SOCIAL MEDIA-INDUCED ANXIETY IN ADOLESCENTS

Considering engagement with social media is virtually inevitable, it is imperative for youth to learn healthy social media habits through self-management strategies. This section explores various strategies for fostering a healthier relationship with social media and promote positive mental well-being for youth living in the digital era.

Establishing Healthy Screen and Social Media Habits

Setting screen time limits

Studies indicate that extended screen time is associated with unhealthy lifestyle habits such as being sedentary, increased junk food consumption, poor sleep, reduced time outdoors, and limited sunlight exposure (summarized in Glover and colleagues[41]). As such, the Office of the US Surgeon General recommends individuals, especially adolescents who are at a crucial physiologic growth stage, establish a daily screen usage limit.[10] The time limit should clearly distinguish between education and recreational screen use including social media interactions. This recommendation is consistent with the results of a recent study on 230 undergraduate students from a university in the Midwestern United States.[42] Findings indicated that limiting social media use to approximately 30 minutes per day resulted in significant improvement in mental health, including a reduction in anxiety, depression, and FOMO.[42]

Limiting screen use before bedtime

Sufficient quality sleep is related to mental and physical well-being and can improve mood and cognitive performance. The blue light emitted by digital devices suppresses the natural nighttime release of melatonin, a hormone that causes drowsiness. Using screens within an hour of bedtime can disrupt natural sleep cycles and adversely impact sleep quality. Browsing social media feeds before sleep may induce over-thinking and ruminations resulting in increased arousal and anxiety that can impair sleep. Youth should be encouraged to cease screen use at least an hour before bedtime, and to engage in calming activities like reading for enjoyment, breathing exercises and meditation to promote better sleep. Youth should also avoid using screen media in bed to avoid deconditioning one's connection with the bed as a place only for sleep.

Periodically practicing "digital detox"

Although this is a new area of study and results have mixed findings,[43] taking intentional prolonged breaks from online entertainment, including social media, has been recommended as an approach to achieve more "balanced" digital habits. A cross-sectional study of 68 university students in Lebanon observed that majority of participants who temporarily abstained from social media activity reported mood improvement, decreased anxiety, and better sleep quality during and immediately following the offline break.[44] Individuals also tended to replace online engagements with in-person social activities during the digital detoxing period.[44] Such periodic offline experiences can promote a more conscious and intentional approach to technology and social media use, and a time to recalibrate, focus, and reset priorities.[45]

Building a Supportive Social Media Environment

Cultivating positive online connections

Nurturing positive online connections is pivotal for youth who use social media.[14] Encouraging healthy online friendships and supportive group dynamics can foster a positive community which may mitigate the negative effects of social media. Being selective about the types of social media platforms used is also important. Choosing platforms that facilitate positive interactions and connection while avoiding those that contribute to anxiety or stress (eg, platforms which foster abusive behavior by allowing users to make public statements while remaining anonymous) can nurture mental well-being.

Recognizing and managing negative thoughts related to social media experiences

Repetitive negative thought patterns attributed to social media experiences can be detrimental to well-being. For example, FOMO and social comparisons can contribute to an adolescent's negative thoughts about themselves and their self-worth. Strategies such as using social media actively (instead of passively scrolling through posts), using social media purposefully and for prescribed periods of time, setting boundaries with peers (eg, "I don't respond to messages after 10 PM"), and prioritizing authentic or in-person interactions could help counteract negative thoughts. Adolescents can develop emotional regulation skills under the guidance of parents and mental health professionals. Seeking support from friends, family, and/or mental health professionals offers valuable perspectives and coping strategies to navigate the complexities of social media-induced emotions.

Oversight at Home: What Can Parents and Caregivers Do?

Parents' screen and social media habits

Parents and caregivers can model healthy digital habits for their children by limiting their own social media and screen use. This may include taking digital breaks, putting their devices out of access before bed and during dinner and other family times, and replacing social media connections with in-person socializing and spending time outdoors. A combination of these efforts reinforces the message that quality family time and in-person interaction is prioritized alongside social media. Parents and caregivers can openly discuss their own experiences with social media by sharing both negative and positive aspects. Such conversations could build trust, encourage children to share their own experiences, and facilitate productive discussions on ways to navigate complex social dynamics that arise on social media.

Managing social media exposure and screen use

Parents and caregivers should set clear guidelines for social media use that are tailored to each child's maturity. New users are encouraged to use a single social media platform to understand its navigation and social dynamics before expanding into others. Children and teens should have a clear understanding of their parents' guidelines and expectations for screen time and social media use as well as potential consequences for misuse. Parents and caregivers should follow their children's social media accounts or designate a trusted adult or sibling to provide oversight. Software exerting parental control can be helpful in both restricting and monitoring online activities, although no type of supervision can fully protect against the evasion of technology savvy, motivated youth. Beginning with close supervision and tight restrictions, which gradually relax as youth demonstrate responsible social media use, is recommended.

Establishing social media communication do's and don'ts

Each family should develop their own set of expectations and guidelines around social media use to reflect the needs and values of family. A written document could be posted in a common area. This document should include the consequences for rule violations. Signing a social media contract can also be considered. It is important that all members of the family are involved in the discussion and in agreement with these guidelines prior to implementation. Other recommendations of social media etiquettes that parents can use as points of discussions are listed in **Table 1**. The AAP has a family media plan template that can be tailored for kids and teens (see link on **Table 2**).

Table 1	
Tips for parents and caregivers pertaining to general do's and don'ts of social media that can serve as discussion points when discussing this topic with their children	
Do's of Social Media	**Don'ts of Social Media**
Stop and think before you post on social media	Do not share personal or identifying information online
Know that everything you post is public and permanent even if it "disappears"	Do not post or send anything you are embarrassed for everyone to see
Make your social media account private, and monitor your privacy settings periodically	
Be kind and respectful on social media	Do not bully or post mean comments online
Set limits on social media and give yourself breaks throughout the day	Do not use social media during family meals, in bed, after bedtime or during class
Prioritize friendships offline and get together with friends in person regularly	Do not neglect in-person socializing for social media
Know that your self-worth is not defined by the number of likes or followers	
Remember that posts on social media are curated and often do not reflect reality	Do not believe that all contents posted in social media are true
Seek help or advise from trusted adult, if you are being bullied online, asked to do something that makes you uncomfortable, or you see a post which makes you think someone could be in danger	
Turn off social media notifications to limit distractions	
Unfollow accounts or people that make you unhappy or feeling badly about yourself	

Table 2
Resources that clinicians can share with youth patients and their parents

Resource	Link to the Resource	Its Potential Use
Facts for Families Guide by the American Academy of Child & Adolescent Psychiatry (AACAP)	Facts For Families (aacap.org)	Downloadable materials to guide families in matters related to youth anxiety and digital media use, such as "Anxiety and Children", "Internet Use in Children", "Screen Time and Children", "Social Media and Teens", and "Video Games and Children: Playing with Violence"
AACAP Screen Media Resource Center	Screen Media Resource Center (aacap.org)	Resources and materials for families around screen media
AAP Center of Excellence on Social Media and Youth Mental Health	https://www.aap.org/en/patient-care/media-and-children/center-of-excellence-on-social-media-and-youth-mental-health/	Resources and materials for providers, families, and policy makers for evidence-based education to support youth navigating social media
American Academy of Pediatrics (AAP) Social Media and Youth Mental Health Q & A Portal	Social Media and Youth Mental Health Q&A Portal (aap.org)	Site to seek answers to questions about social medial and youth mental health
HealthyChildren.org website by the American Academy of Pediatrics (AAP)	https://www.healthychildren.org/English/family-life/Media/ AND https://www.healthychildren.org/English/fmp/Pages/MediaPlan.aspx	Practical guidelines and support for families around youth digital media use including the ability to create a customizable family media plan
Age-based Media Reviews for Families by Common Sense Media	https://www.commonsensemedia.org/	Parent-focused and educator-focused youth digital media guide with age-based ratings of appropriateness of games, apps, and YouTube channels
Protecting Youth Mental Health, U.S. Surgeon General's Advisory, 2021	https://www.hhs.gov/surgeongeneral/priorities/youth-mental-health/index.html	Advisory document and action items for youth mental health with significant sections on youth anxiety and social media and video game companies' responsibilities
Social Media and Youth Mental Health, U.S. Surgeon General's Advisory, 2023	https://www.hhs.gov/surgeongeneral/priorities/youth-mental-health/social-media/index.html	Describes current evidence on the impacts of social media on youth mental health
AACAP Policy Statement on Impact of Social Media and Youth Mental Health	Policy Statement on the Impact of Social Media on Youth Mental Health (aacap.org)	

(continued on next page)

Table 2 (continued)		
Resource	Link to the Resource	Its Potential Use
Teens and Tech Research Compilation by the Winston National Center on Technology Use, Brain, and Psychological Development	https://www.teensandtech. org/	Adolescent, researcher, and clinician guides for a more detailed, research analysis on brain development as related to digital media use
Children and Screens (part of the Institute of Digital Media and Child Development)	https://www. childrenandscreens.org/	An institution that offers a wide range of interdisciplinary research and current information on digital media and child development
Cyberbullying Research Center	https://cyberbullying.org/	An organization that provides pertinent and current information about cyberbullying among adolescents, including news, personal stories, facts and figures, guidelines, and others
Screen Sanity	https://screensanity.org/	A non-profit organization that offers tips, tools, and training for parents to help families maximize technology's benefits while minimizing potential harm

Cultivating a healthy digital culture in the family

It is important that families work together to cultivate a healthy digital culture at home. This may include all members putting smartphones away during family time including at meals, movie nights, or family games. Parents should consider setting an example by following many or all of the same rules they set for their children. A common area in the home for charging smartphones can be helpful to keep devices out of the bedrooms.

Establishing an open communication practice with their children

Caregivers should establish open and honest conversations with their children about social media usage. Creating a safe space and practicing active listening encourage youth to share their experiences. This is facilitated by parents taking a curious, nonjudgmental attitude when their children's share social media experiences, and resisting restriction of the child's phone when the child shares something concerning. It is equally crucial for parents to watch for and investigate any changes in their children's behavior, such as alterations in mood, sleep, academic performance, appearance and body image, preoccupation with certain thoughts, and excessive worries. Concerns raised by children about FOMO, online comparisons, or social media interactions should be explored to foster healthy decisions regarding social media. If parents feel unable to help their children with such issues, they should consider referral to a qualified mental health specialist.

Clinical Oversight: What Can Health Care Professionals Do?

Recent systematic, narrative, and scoping reviews recognize the association of social media with anxiety and depression in adolescents.[15,17,41,46] These reviews collectively emphasize the crucial role of health care providers (eg, pediatricians, primary care providers, child psychiatrists, and therapists) in screening for social media use and online engagement during well-child visits. Routine inquiries about social media involvement, platforms, usage patterns, and emotional impact should be integrated into patient assessments. This allows clinicians to learn about the social media profiles and virtual activities of young patients, which potentially could lead to active discussions about their social media habits. Some patients may also share their social media feed with providers if asked, which can be very informative regarding what type of content is typically viewed. Health care visits can also facilitate conversations between youth and their caregivers regarding appropriate social media etiquette and habits. This approach may enable addressing any potential social media-induced anxiety in teenagers and facilitate needed family communication.

When social media habits or experiences contribute to anxiety, sleep disturbance, negative body image, and/or poor self-esteem, clinicians should offer strategies to address these concerns. These recommendations may include setting time limits for screen and social media usage, helping youth block "triggering" content from their social media feed, offering opportunities for alternative activities with friends and family, and other strategies outlined in previous sections. Incorporating techniques from cognitive behavioral therapy (CBT) such as reframing distorted or overvalued thoughts, creating alternative activity options in place of engaging in social media, and conducting therapeutic exposures (eg, refraining from checking social media, turning of notifications, and banning the phone from the bedroom) can also be effective.[47] If these strategies are insufficient to alleviate anxiety and other mental health issues, then referral to a mental health professional is advised. Medications can also be considered for severe cases in which compulsive social media use causes impairment of daily functioning. **Table 2** provides various resources that clinicians can share with youth patients and their parents.

CASE STUDY
Case 1

L.K. was a 9 year old fourth grader admitted for inpatient psychiatric care due to increased aggression, suicidal and homicidal ideation, which appear related to having been relocated from rural South Dakota to Nebraska a month prior. During the admission interview, L.K. proudly reported he had a YouTube channel with 71 "subs" (subscribers). Upon additional inquiry, he admitted to posing as a 23 year old to register his channel. L.K. reported that the move was hard for him, and he was only beginning to make new friends in the new school. His psychiatric review noted excessive worry, school anxiety, and symptoms of attention-deficit/hyperactivity disorder. His mother knew about his YouTube channel, but not his stated age. She had viewed many of his posts, which showed L.K. dancing and singing, and presenting various homages to Michael Jackson. In recent months, when restricted from YouTube and online access, L.K. exhibited dysregulation, verbal and physical aggression, and expressed a sense of futility of life. L.K.'s mother found setting limits on her son's technology usage increasingly challenging due to his severe reactions.

Review of Case 1

This case typifies preadolescent exposure to and engagement in social media. L.K.'s YouTube channel gave him a sense of mastery, pride, and means to connect with others during a lonely time of transition. His falsified age placed him in a category free from appropriate restrictions or safeguards. L.K.'s mother was unaware of this lapse despite taking appropriate steps to monitor his social media content. L.K.'s explosive response to limit-setting could be a manifestation of an addictive quality of his social media use leading to extreme anxiety at the thought of not having access or withdrawal. His clinicians recommended a higher level of social media supervision and reducing parental accommodation to screen use through family psychoeducation on extinction bursts. Family members were also encouraged to develop mindfulness activities to alleviate anxiety, as well as to incorporate a family media use plan (HealthyChildren.org, website by the AAP; **Table 2**).

Case 2

S.D. was a 15 year old girl presenting concerns of anxiety and self-harm via cutting. According to her parents, S.D.'s diary entries described feelings of loneliness and peer exclusion. She described upward comparisons by finding peers to be more accomplished, smarter, and more attractive. S.D. conveyed self-loathing and poor self-esteem ("*I feel like I have no place or purpose here*"). Her parents indicated that S.D. was previously "*a bubbly, outgoing and social kid.*" Upon entering middle school, she developed social anxiety and difficulty making friends, although these situations appeared to partially resolve. The COVID-19 pandemic caused another disruption to her social life, and upon entering high school in person, she once again struggled to fit in the new social milieu. Perceiving social cliques as barriers to making new friends, she withdrew and started spending extended hours on her phone to scroll through social media or watch YouTube and avoiding social opportunities like extracurricular activities.

In her clinical assessment, S.D. expressed being excluded and feeling self-conscious when interacting with others, fearing she might appear awkward or boring. She observed social media posts of peers socializing with some degree of envy and self-doubt ("*I don't know what to say and they seem like they have more interesting and fun lives. I feel like I am boring, and they would not want to hang out with me.*"). When asked about her social media use, S.D. reported closely following the posts of her peers, but refrained from commenting or making her own posts. She continued to devote much of her free time to passive social media use despite the intensified loneliness it instilled in her. The constant exposure to peers' apparent success heightened her sense of missing out, resulting in ever-more frequent checking of posts. Her compulsive checking, conducted even before bed and during class, further exacerbated her isolation. Persistent worry about life, the future, and loneliness also gradually undermined her sleep quality.

Review of Case 2

This case underscores how teen social media use can trigger FOMO and exacerbate social anxiety and low self-esteem. S.D.'s self-comparison to the cultivated social media posts of her peers eroded her self-esteem, which exacerbated her self-consciousness, leading to avoidance of initiating social interactions and preventing new friendships. Her social media habit created a distorted perception of her peers, leading her to believe they were more interesting and secure in established social groups. Guidance in developing a more realistic appraisal of her peers and fostering healthier self-esteem could provide the confidence to initiate and sustain positive online relationships, which could eventually lead to a more fulfilling and frequent in-person interactions.

NAVIGATING A NEW DIGITAL ERA: IT IS AN EVOLVING FIELD

Smartphones and other computer screens play an integral part of contemporary life, serving as vital vehicles that deliver various modes of entertainment, learning, and communication. Social media platforms are increasingly embedded into the fabric of our society. Social media has also transformed into a diverse, albeit often unreliable, platform for information shared by countless individuals within the vast virtual community. In this way, open access to and pervasive engagement with social media can significantly influence the way youth understand and navigate the world.

This article is conceived, written, and published, in a time of unprecedented concern regarding the impact of social media on youth mental health, as expressed on the international, national, and state levels. Legislative hearings are conducted where lawmakers question social media experts and executives to inform the development of guidelines and policies governing technology development and platform usage.[48,49] There is also an ongoing public discussion about the youth mental health crisis that is focusing on potential school- or community-based programs and interventions for preventing and treating mental illness among youth.[50] Pertinent questions raised during the discussion include "should socioemotional educational activities include social media and digital technology literacy?", and "how should parents and caregivers alter their own social media practices and support their children's journey into the digital world?". Public opinion about these issues and related legal and cultural consequences will largely determine how youth interact with social media going forward, with massive implications for their future well-being. Pediatric providers must keep abreast of such changes to best advise families and treat children whose lives are impacted regularly by social media.

CLINICS CARE POINTS

- There is growing evidence linking social media use to increased anxiety among youth and teens.
- At annual well care visits, primary care providers should consider assessing screen time and social media use, and initiating discussion about this topic with youth and their parents.
- Children and teens should be informed about the impact of social media habits and online experiences on their well-being, to achieve healthy, balanced lives. Parental and school-imposed restrictions on social media access could also be applied when necessary.
- Incorporating techniques from CBT such as reframing thoughts, distractions, exposure therapy (eg, avoiding checking and refreshing social media feeds), among others can be effective for treatment of youth with social media overuse and anxiety.

DISCLOSURE

All authors declare that they have no conflict of interest.

REFERENCES

1. Petrosyan A. Worlwide digital population. Statista 2024. Available at: https://www.statista.com/statistics/617136/digital-population-worldwide/.
2. Jones M. The complete history of social media: a timeline of the invention of online networking. History Cooperative 2024. Available at: https://historycooperative.org/the-history-of-social-media/. Accessed February 15, 2024.
3. "Social media". In Merriam-Webster.com dictionary, Merriam-Webster. Retrieved 2 February 2024.

4. Anderson M, Faverio M, Gottfried J. Teens, social media and technology 2023. 2023. Available at: https://www.pewresearch.org/internet/2023/12/11/teens-social-media-and-technology-2023/. Accessed December 11, 2023.

5. Rideout V. The common sense census: Media use by kids age zero to eight in America, A Common Sense Media Research study. Inter-University Consortium for Political and Social Research (distributor). 2021. https://doi.org/10.3886/ICPSR37491.v2.

6. Rideout V, Peebles A, Mann S, et al. Common sense census: media use by tweens and teens, 2021. 2022. Available at: https://www.commonsensemedia.org/research/the-common-sense-census-media-use-by-tweens-and-teens-2021.

7. Kessler RC, Berglund P, Demler O, et al. Lifetime prevalence and age-of-onset distributions of dsm-iv disorders in the national comorbidity survey replication. Arch Gen Psychiatr 2005;62(6):593–602.

8. Beesdo K, Knappe S, Pine DS. Anxiety and anxiety disorders in children and adolescents: developmental issues and implications for dsm-v. Psychiatr Clin 2009; 32(3):483–524.

9. Lebrun-Harris LA, Ghandour RM, Kogan MD, et al. Five-year trends in us children's health and well-being, 2016-2020. JAMA Pediatr 2022;176(7):e220056. https://doi.org/10.1001/jamapediatrics.2022.0056.

10. Office of the Surgeon General (OSG). Protecting youth mental health: the U.S. Surgeon General's Advisory. Publications and Reports of the Surgeon General; 2021.

11. AAP, AACAP, CHA declare national emergency in children's mental health. 2021. Available at: https://publications.aap.org/aapnews/news/17718?autologincheck=redirected. Accessed February 10, 2023.

12. Orben A, Przybylski AK, Blakemore SJ, et al. Windows of developmental sensitivity to social media. Nat Commun 2022;13(1):1649.

13. Wang H, Zhao J, Yu Z, et al. Types of on-screen content and mental health in kindergarten children. JAMA Pediatr 2024;178(2):125–32.

14. Office of the Surgeon General (OSG). Social media and youth mental health. Publications and Reports of the Surgeon General. 2023. Available at: https://www.hhs.gov/sites/default/files/sg-youth-mental-health-social-media-advisory.pdf.

15. Hilty DM, Stubbe D, McKean AJ, et al. A scoping review of social media in child, adolescents and young adults: research findings in depression, anxiety and other clinical challenges. BJPsych Open 2023;9(5):e152.

16. Lai F, Wang L, Zhang J, et al. Relationship between social media use and social anxiety in college students: mediation effect of communication capacity. Int J Environ Res Publ Health 2023;20(4). https://doi.org/10.3390/ijerph20043657.

17. Prasad S, Ait Souabni S, Anugwom G, et al. Anxiety and depression amongst youth as adverse effects of using social media : a review. Ann Med Surg (Lond) 2023;85(8):3974–81.

18. Gingras MP, Brendgen M, Beauchamp MH, et al. Adolescents and social media: longitudinal links between types of use, problematic use and internalizing symptoms. Res Child Adolesc Psychopathol 2023;51(11):1641–55.

19. Maza MT, Fox KA, Kwon SJ, et al. Association of habitual checking behaviors on social media with longitudinal functional brain development. JAMA Pediatr 2023; 177(2):160–7.

20. Jiang S, Ngien A. The effects of instagram use, social comparison, and self-esteem on social anxiety: a survey study in Singapore. Social Media Society 2020;6(2). https://doi.org/10.1177/2056305120912488. 2056305120912488.

21. Muqaddas J, Sanobia Anwwer S, Nawaz A. Impact of social media on self-esteem. European Scientific Journal, ESJ 2017;13(23). https://doi.org/10.19044/esj.2017.v13n23p329.

22. McCarthy PA, Morina N. Exploring the association of social comparison with depression and anxiety: a systematic review and meta-analysis. Clin Psychol Psychother 2020;27(5):640–71.

23. Tiraboschi GA, Garon-Carrier G, Smith J, et al. Adolescent internet use predicts higher levels of generalized and social anxiety symptoms for girls but not boys. Prev Med Rep 2023;36:102471.

24. Plackett R, Sheringham J, Dykxhoorn J. The longitudinal impact of social media use on UK adolescents' mental health: longitudinal observational study. J Med Internet Res 2023;25:e43213.

25. Seekis V, Kennedy R. The impact of #beauty and #self-compassion tiktok videos on young women's appearance shame and anxiety, self-compassion, mood, and comparison processes. Body Image 2023;45:117–25.

26. Laughter MR, Anderson JB, Maymone MBC, et al. Psychology of aesthetics: beauty, social media, and body dysmorphic disorder. Clin Dermatol 2023; 41(1):28–32.

27. Angelini F, Gini G. Differences in perceived online communication and disclosing e-motions among adolescents and young adults: the role of specific social media features and social anxiety. J Adolesc 2023. https://doi.org/10.1002/jad.12256.

28. Notara V, Vagka E, Gnardellis C, et al. The emerging phenomenon of nomophobia in young adults: a systematic review study. Addict Health 2021;13(2):120–36.

29. Hisler GC, Hasler BP, Franzen PL, et al. Screen media use and sleep disturbance symptom severity in children. Sleep Health 2020;6(6):731–42.

30. Franchina V, Vanden Abeele M, van Rooij AJ, et al. Fear of missing out as a predictor of problematic social media use and phubbing behavior among Flemish adolescents. Int J Environ Res Publ Health 2018;15(10). https://doi.org/10.3390/ijerph15102319.

31. Papapanou TK, Darviri C, Kanaka-Gantenbein C, et al. Strong correlations between social appearance anxiety, use of social media, and feelings of loneliness in adolescents and young adults. Int J Environ Res Publ Health 2023;20(5). https://doi.org/10.3390/ijerph20054296.

32. Gupta M, Sharma A. Fear of missing out: a brief overview of origin, theoretical underpinnings and relationship with mental health. World J Clin Cases 2021;9(19): 4881–9.

33. Anto A, Asif RO, Basu A, et al. Exploring the impact of social media on anxiety among university students in the United Kingdom: qualitative study. JMIR Form Res 2023;7:e43037.

34. Scott H, Woods HC. Fear of missing out and sleep: cognitive behavioural factors in adolescents' nighttime social media use. J Adolesc 2018;68:61–5.

35. Starvaggi I, Dierckman C, Lorenzo-Luaces L. Mental health misinformation on social media: review and future directions. Curr Opin Psychol 2023;56:101738. https://doi.org/10.1016/j.copsyc.2023.101738.

36. Gupta R, Ariefdjohan M. Mental illness on instagram: a mixed method study to characterize public content, sentiments, and trends of antidepressant use. J Ment Health 2020;1–8. https://doi.org/10.1080/09638237.2020.1755021.

37. McMullan RD, Berle D, Arnáez S, et al. The relationships between health anxiety, online health information seeking, and cyberchondria: systematic review and meta-analysis. J Affect Disord 2019;245:270–8.

38. Starcevic V. Cyberchondria: challenges of problematic online searches for health-related information. Psychother Psychosom 2017;86(3):129–33.
39. Chochol MD, Gandhi K, Elmaghraby R, et al. Harnessing youth engagement with mental health tiktok and its potential as a public health tool. J Am Acad Child Adolesc Psychiatry 2023;62(7):710–2.
40. Abu Khait A, Mrayyan MT, Al-Rjoub S, et al. Cyberchondria, anxiety sensitivity, hypochondria, and internet addiction: implications for mental health professionals. Curr Psychol 2022;1–12. https://doi.org/10.1007/s12144-022-03815-3.
41. Glover J, Ariefdjohan M, Fritsch SL. #kidsanxiety and the digital world. Child Adolesc Psychiatr Clin N Am 2022;31(1):71–90.
42. Faulhaber ME, Lee JE, Gentile DA. The effect of self-monitoring limited social media use on psychological well-being. Technology, Mind, and Behavior 2023;4(2). https://doi.org/10.1037/tmb0000111.
43. Radtke T, Apel T, Schenkel K, et al. Digital detox: an effective solution in the smartphone era? A systematic literature review. Mob Media Commun 2022; 10(2):190–215.
44. El-Khoury J, Haidar R, Kanj RR, et al. Characteristics of social media 'detoxification' in university students. Libyan J Med 2021;16(1):1846861.
45. Schmuck D. Does digital detox work? Exploring the role of digital detox applications for problematic smartphone use and well-being of young adults using multi-group analysis. Cyberpsychol, Behav Soc Netw 2020;23(8):526–32.
46. Chochol MD, Gandhi K, Croarkin PE. Social media and anxiety in youth: a narrative review and clinical update. Child Adolesc Psychiatr Clin N Am 2023;32(3): 613–30.
47. Alutaybi A, Al-Thani D, McAlaney J, et al. Combating fear of missing out (fomo) on social media: the fomo-r method. Int J Environ Res Publ Health 2020;17(17). https://doi.org/10.3390/ijerph17176128.
48. Isaac M. Six takeaways from a contentious online child safety hearing. The New York Times 2024. Available at: https://www.nytimes.com/2024/01/31/technology/tech-senate-hearing-child-safety.html?unlocked_article_code=1.SE0.JaUZ. Yz72mwXGnr1T&bgrp=a&smid=url-share. Accessed February 2, 2024.
49. Kang C, McCabe D. 'Your product is killing people': tech leaders denounced over child safety. The New York Times 2024. Available at: https://www.nytimes.com/2024/01/31/technology/senate-child-safety-social-media.html?unlocked_article_code=1.SE0.g8O8.ZvaZslrr6mp6&bgrp=a&smid=url-share. Accessed February 2, 2024.
50. Anderer S. Social media industry standards needed to protect adolescent mental health, says national academies. JAMA 2024. https://doi.org/10.1001/jama.2023.28259.

Cyberbullying and Online Aggression

Jennifer L. Yen, MD[a,b,*,1], Christopher Chamanadjian, MD[c,2]

KEYWORDS

- Cyberbullying • Cybervictimization • Cyberstalking • Problematic social media use
- Problematic internet use

KEY POINTS

- Cyberbullying has been identified as a public health issue among children and adolescents.
- Definitions of cyberbullying vary depending on the study but all include the use of technology to carry out an intentional act of aggression and/or harm to another.
- Risk factors for cyberbullying victims and perpetrators include gender, age, socioeconomic status, and excessive or problematic social media use.
- Cyberbullying has a significant negative impact on both victims and perpetrators, resulting in deterioration in physical and mental health.
- Prevention programs, particularly in a school setting, show promise as potential interventions to reduce cyberbullying and mitigate negative consequences.

INTRODUCTION

As digital technology advances allow for easier access to the Internet, youth are spending more and more time online. This was amplified by the coronavirus disease 2019 (COVID-19) pandemic, during which social distancing and virtual classes increased screen time for all children and adolescents. In many cases, youth are engaging with popular social media (SM) platforms such as Instagram, Snapchat, TikTok, YouTube, and Facebook to communicate and connect with peers. According to Pew Research Center, about 24% of teens in their 2014 to 2015 survey reported "almost constant" Internet use. By 2023, 46% of teens had reported the same amount of time spent.

Minoritized teens spend more time than their White counterparts, as do those with lower socioeconomic status (SES). Girls spend more time on SM, while boys are more

^a Department of Psychiatry and Behavioral Sciences, Baylor College of Medicine, Houston, TX, USA; ^b The Harris Center for Mental Health and IDD, Houston, TX, USA; ^c Department of Psychiatry, Charles R. Drew University of Medicine and Science, CA, USA
¹ Present address: 2400 McCue Road #425, Houston, TX 77056.
² Present address: 1635 Malcolm Ave, Los Angeles, CA 90024.
* Corresponding author. PO Box 27208, Houston, TX 77227.
E-mail address: jlyenmd@gmail.com

Pediatr Clin N Am 72 (2025) 333–349
https://doi.org/10.1016/j.pcl.2024.09.004   **pediatric.theclinics.com**

likely to use streaming platforms.[1] With youth having access to the Internet through various forms of technology—smartphones, tablets, desktop and laptop computers, and gaming consoles—excessive screen use and problematic behaviors have since been identified. One such area of concern is cyberbullying.

While traditional bullying is well recognized as having a harmful impact on youth mental health, cyberbullying has grown into a major issue. One of the first documented cases occurred in 1998 in Pennsylvania, where the state Supreme Court ruled to uphold the school expulsion of the 14 year old perpetrator.[2] Over the years, more cases have been brought to public attention, particularly those involving deaths by suicide that occurred after experiencing cyberbullying.

Though now a widely recognized phenomenon, research into the topic is still relatively new. Most of the studies on cyberbullying have occurred from 2007 to 2020, with inconsistent, sometimes contradictory, results.[3] Nonetheless, all of them agree that the negative impact cyberbullying has on the victims is significant and persistent, with deteriorations in both mental and physical health. As such, the Centers for Disease Control and Prevention (CDC) has deemed it a serious public health threat and provided warnings and safeguards to the public at large.[4]

DEFINITIONS

One of the major factors contributing to the lack of consistent information on cyberbullying is its definition. The CDC refers to cyberbullying as "electronic aggression," defining it as "any type of harassment or bullying that occurs through e-mail, a chat room, instant messaging, a Web site (including blogs), or text messaging."[4]

Other terms utilized by scholars include "cyberstalking," "online aggression," "cyber harassment," "Internet harassment," "Internet bullying," and "cyber victimization."[5]

Each identifies a specific aspect of cyberbullying, including

- The use of technology
- The intention to harm
- The hostile nature of the act
- Repetition over time

However, repetition can be indirect or unintentional, such as when a single act shared by a larger group achieves viral status due to its content or identified victim. Alternately, given the lack of understanding many youths have regarding the permanence of online information, past acts may re-emerge at a later point, resulting in renewed harm.

As such, Tokunaga suggested a more encompassing definition, describing cyberbullying as "any behavior performed through electronic or digital media by individuals or groups that repeatedly communicates hostile or aggressive messages intended to inflict harm or discomfort on others."[6,7]

Other research has raised the concept of power imbalance, suggesting that a disparity between victim and perpetrator is a crucial component of cyberbullying.[8] When combined with cultural factors, the definition of cyberbullying becomes more complex, as differences appear in what is considered aggressive behavior, and the terms used to describe it, vary among countries and cultures.[9]

PREVALENCE

Prevalence rates for cyberbullying, like its definition, have been difficult to ascertain. Rates of victimization vary by country, gender, and age group. For studies that considered victimization, perpetration, or both, it was found that between 4% and 72% of children and adolescents were affected. Much of the variation is attributed to the lack of a consistent definition, the difference in methodologies, and the heterogeneity of the study samples.[5] Another potential reason for the variation is the willingness of victims and perpetrators to report cyberbullying. The former might avoid doing so over fear of their parents removing their technology, retaliation by the perpetrator, or embarrassment over being victimized. Perpetrators are likely to underreport to avoid consequences or prevent themselves from being seen in a negative light.[5] In addition, cyberbullying acts are easier to hide and trace, resulting in underestimation of true prevalence. However, the majority of studies conducted estimates the rates of cyberbullying victimization to be around 20% to 40%.[6,7,10]

A recent study by Nagata and colleagues[11] looked at the social epidemiology of cyberbullying in early adolescence. Their study of 9429 ethnically diverse 11 to 12 year olds found a lifetime prevalence of cyberbullying victimization of 9.6%, with 65.8% occurring in the past 12 months. Lifetime prevalence of perpetration was 1.1%, with 59.8% occurring in the past 12 months. Their conclusion was that 1 in 10 early adolescents had already experienced cyberbullying victimization in their lifetime.

When evaluating cyberbullying around the world, prevalence rates also vary widely. Studies conducted in European countries on 14 to 17 year old adolescents, specifically Romania, Greece, Germany, and Poland, revealed rates between 21.5% and 37.3%.[12] In Spain, a study of 9 to 18 year olds reported 25.1% as victims, while 3.9% were reported as perpetrators.[13] A study in South Korea of 4000 students' grades 7 to 12 found 14.6% were victims and 6.3% were perpetrators.[14] In contrast, a study of 102 Indonesian 12 to 13 year old students found 80% reported being victimized sometime in their life.[15]

TYPES OF CYBERBULLYING

While its exact definition is still up for debate, cyberbullying can be separated into several distinctive types that distinguish it from traditional physical bullying.[16]

1. Flaming—angry or vulgar messages
2. Harassment—consistent stream of offensive messages
3. Denigration—damaging messages about the victim are sent to those known to them
4. Masquerading—stealing victim's identity to create harmful or damaging messages
5. Trickery—deceiving the victim for personal or financial information
6. Exclusion—ostracization from a social group
7. Stalking—obtaining personal information from SM profiles (such as location or associates) or hacking
8. Blackmailing—using anonymous emails, phone calls, and private messages to solicit money or actions from the victim

Additionally, studies by Palasinski and others[17] include a ninth type, "happy slapping," in which traditional bullying meets cyberbullying through a victim being subjected to various forms of violence as humiliation and recorded on video for posting online.[18]

Some scholars argue certain forms of harassment should be viewed in a distinctive and separate light. Copp and colleagues[19] note that some definitions of cyberbullying include behaviors that constitute sexual harassment, such as sending unwanted sexual content or asking someone to do something sexual. However, as sexual harassment is recognized as a form of gender-based violence, they suggest online sexual harassment should be independently studied for prevalence, risk factors, and potential consequences and viewed somewhat separately from other forms of cyberbullying.

In many cases, what may start out as one form of cyberbullying will evolve to include the others. An example can be a perpetrator initially stalking their victim's SM profiles looking for damaging information, and then utilizing it to blackmail, flame, and denigrate them.

CAUSES AND CONTRIBUTING FACTORS

While many theories have been put forth regarding potential causal factors of cyberbullying, problematic SM use is one of the most strongly and consistently associated for both victimization and perpetration. A study by Craig and colleagues[20] utilized contemporary social theories to provide frameworks to link problematic SM use to cyberbullying, including

1. Frequent and intense SM use exposes adolescents to aggressive behavior, including cyberbullying
2. Repeated exposure to online aggression can normalize and make the behavior seem more acceptable through role modeling and reinforcement
3. Witnessing social rewards of aggression or cyberbullying (increased status) reinforces behavior and conforming to group norms
4. Lack of face-to-face cues hides negative consequences, encouraging repetition of acts[20]

A study by Ho and colleagues[21] suggests that the leading factors for perpetration are the presence of normative thinking, involvement in aggressive peer groups, and peer pressure. In addition, youth with low self-control and difficulty with moral identity are more vulnerable to being influenced. As their peer group normalizes aggressive behavior, including cyberbullying, the youth will then view the behavior as acceptable even if it contradicts known values.

Additionally, there are several other factors that have been posited as contributing to cyberbullying. The first is anonymity. Digital technology and SM platforms allow for perpetrators to hide their identity through fake profiles or throwaway accounts. They can also, as previously mentioned, masquerade as someone else (ie, the victim) by hacking into their account or creating a new one. Many times, youth perpetrators believe deactivating or simply deleting their posts or messages will prevent them from being discovered or held responsible. The lack of immediate, visible reaction from their victim also enforces the perpetrator's disinhibition.[22]

While more research needs to be completed on the effect of poor interpersonal relationships in cyberbullying, one study associated lack of parental involvement and communication as contributing to increased occurrences.[23] For victims, the lack of support makes them more vulnerable to attack, as they may suffer from loneliness, anxiety, or depression, and do not have the coping mechanisms to handle personal attacks. For perpetrators, the lack of monitoring generates more opportunities to offend, and cyberbullying may serve as an outlet for unresolved anger and aggression toward the parents or others.

A review conducted by Santre[8] also points at social dominance theory as a potential contributor. The theory proposes people belong either to a subordinate group or to a dominant group. Two types of behavior will determine one's peer group rank: those that increase social prominence and those that increase social dominance (control and power). Much the same as traditional bullying, cyberbullying can be used to obtain or sustain a higher rank in the social group. This is often seen with more popular or rebellious youth. The former may utilize it to exercise control over their friend group and eliminate competition, and the latter to incite fear in those they feel judge them and generate an "infamous" persona.

Meanwhile, causal factors for victimization include individual behavior, sense of self, and the environment. Many youths who prefer digital communication may also be from more vulnerable backgrounds, including those with psychosocial issues. Being online excessively may positively affect their mood, but the lack of social resources and skills to defend themselves puts them at risk of being victimized. Studies looking into the social behaviors of those reporting cyberbullying found an associated tendency to post indiscreet information and content on SM without security.[24] This allows their content to be shared or manipulated without permission, and their profiles or accounts hacked or used for negative gain.

Facial features have also been found to contribute to a higher risk of being cyberbullied. A study by Rudert and colleagues[25] found many ostracized victims were those whose faces were viewed as cold (unfriendly) or incompetent. Though youth who are not conventionally attractive are likely to become targets, those who are considered pretty or handsome may also be victimized by a jealous perpetrator.

CHARACTERISTICS OF CYBERBULLYING VICTIMS AND PERPETRATORS

Though any individual has the potential to become victimized or to perpetrate cyberbullying, some trends have been noted by researchers. In a study conducted by Ybarra and Mitchell[26] using a telephone survey of 1500 individuals aged 10 to 17 years in the United States found that perpetrators often suffered from a wide range of psychosocial issues as well, including mental, social, and behavioral problems. They were noted to be more likely to act aggressively in nature, to engage in rule breaking, complain about parental relationships, and to have themselves experienced victimization both online and offline.

The association between age and cyberbullying is up for debate. In a systematic review conducted by Aboujaoude and colleagues,[5] most studies did not find a significant association, though a few suggested that as the age increased, so did the rate of victimization. The possibility was raised that the rate is nonlinear; in fact, several studies suggest the rate of victimization might be low in childhood, rise in early adolescence, and then fall again when they mature into adulthood. This theory is supported by a study on traditional bullying across late childhood and early adolescence, where the rates declined overall across the transition from primary school to secondary school.[27]

In the study by Nagata,[11] boys reported higher odds of perpetration and lower odds of victimization compared to girls. This gender separation has been confirmed through multiple other studies, revealing that girls are victimized more frequently than boys. Another study suggested adolescent female individuals are victimized at the highest rates, with 18% at the age of 13 years, 15% at the age of 14 years, 24% at the age of 15 years, and 21% at the age of 16 years.[28] This continued in college, where 44% of female students have reported experiencing some degree of cybervictimization.[29] Meanwhile, Craig and colleagues[20] found that girls had higher rates of both perpetration and victimization as it related to their problematic SM use. A higher amount of time spent online, exposure to aggression, and frequent contact with strangers were identified as likely reasons for this finding.

As previously noted, Pew Research Center found that youth in lower SES households spent more time online than their higher SES counterparts.[1] This is supported by a 31 country study by Soares and colleagues,[30] which reported the same increased screen time, leading to greater exposure to cyberbullying and eventual risk of both victimization and perpetration. In the Nagata[11] study, their findings additionally revealed youth from lower household incomes had 1.62 higher odds of cyberbullying than those from higher income households. While none of the studies focused on possible explanations for this disparity, factors could include reduced parental supervision, safety concerns outside the home, and communication problems related to culture or stigma.

Interestingly, the evidence surrounding ethnic minorities and risk of cyberbullying has been mixed. Some studies have pointed at a higher rate of cyberbullying in majority (White) youth, while others have found the opposite. Barlett and Wright[31] found a significant relationship between cyberbullying victimization and perpetration in majority youth only, but not for minoritized youth. However, Kowalski and colleagues[32] reported similar cyberbullying victimization and perpetration behaviors between Black and White respondents in their study. In a 2022 study looking at anti-Asian hate and discrimination against Asian Americans, the prevalence of cyberbullying rose during the COVID-19 pandemic, but mental health outcomes did not differ when compared to their Latinx and White counterparts.[33] Further research is necessary to further examine the impact of ethnic minority status on cyberbullying.

With regards to sexual minority youth, however, the research is clearer. A review of the literature by Abreu and Kenny on LGBTQIA+ youth in 5 countries found that sexual minority and gender expansive youth reported more exposure to anonymous forms of cyberbullying than their heterosexual counterparts. In addition, it is consistently ranked the highest form of prejudice, affecting 28% to 48.95% of sexual minority youth.[34] Other results from their review included

- Students who identified as a sexual minority reported more cyberbullying (9.7%) than traditional bullying (8.2%)
- Sexual minority youth were harassed for both their biological sex and their gender identity or expression
- Cisgender nonheterosexual female individuals, transgender, and youth with "other" genders reported more cyberbullying than cisgender gay and bisexual male individuals
- Bisexual youth may be more susceptible to cyberbullying than other sexual minorities[35]
- Bisexual female students experienced more cyberbullying than lesbian counterparts
- Gay male individuals were more likely to be bullied than bisexual male individuals[36]

Additional studies noted the findings regarding bisexual students may demonstrate a gender difference when it comes to cyberbullying. As with cisgender study findings, race and ethnicity did not seem to significantly impact the rates in this population.

Though limited, some studies have focused on the prevalence and correlates of cyberbullying victimization and perpetration in adolescents and youth adults with disabilities. Kowalski and Toth[37] found that regardless of disability status, the participants reported victimization, with the highest rates among individuals with disabilities, while there was no significant difference for perpetration. In a retrospective study by Nicolai and colleagues,[38] young adults who stuttered and were cyberbullied as adolescents exhibited greater levels of depression and other long-term consequences compared to those who were not victimized.

IMPACT OF CYBERBULLYING ON HEALTH AND WELL-BEING

Regardless of definition or population, all studies found exposure to cyberbullying has significant negative impact on physical and mental well-being. As previously mentioned, perpetrators are often found to have low psychological well-being, struggle with parental relationships, and exhibit increased externalizing behaviors. These negative feelings have been reported as providing moral "justification" for attacking others.[39] One study found comorbidities such as conduct problems, hyperactivity, alcohol use, and tobacco use in cyberbullies.[40] A subset of perpetrators, termed "bully-victims," cyberbully others to deal with their negative emotions or in retaliation to those who harmed them. They have been found to be more troubled than perpetrators or victims, with more interpersonal and conduct problems and higher suicide risk.[10,40]

Multiple studies have shown victims experience significant adverse outcomes from cyberbullying. They may exhibit headaches, disordered eating, weight changes, gastrointestinal distress, and sleep disturbance. This is directly related to the low self-esteem and self-image, avoidant or fearful behavior, depression, and social anxiety they develop from cyberbullying. This in turn leads to low academic performance, substance use, suicidal ideation, and most concerning, suicide attempts.[8,40]

One meta-analysis noted that peer victimization resulted in 2.23 higher odds for suicidal ideation and 2.55 higher odds for suicide attempts.[41] The same analysis revealed that cyberbullying was more strongly linked than traditional bullying to suicidal ideation. These rates are even higher when considering minoritized youth. Duong and Bradshaw[42] found that the risk of attempted suicide was 4.72 times greater for sexual minority youth who had experienced cyberbullying, and those who had been victimized through traditional bullying as well had 8.30 times greater risk. Of additional concern, the review by Santre[8] found suggested linkage of victimization with increased school aggression and higher risk of bringing a weapon to school.

Clinical Case 1

A 13 year old female individual comes to the clinic with a parent for a child and adolescent psychiatry follow-up visit. Parent reports she has missed several days of school and states, "she mostly watches Netflix now and is not on her phone as much."

INTERVIEWING/SCREENING

With the rapidly evolving digital landscape and cyberbullying, a public health issue, it is important for clinicians to recognize a potential victim or perpetrator during evaluation or treatment. This includes a working knowledge of the various technological platforms and tactics used in cyberbullying, such as SM platforms (Facebook, Instagram, X, TikTok, Snapchat, Reddit, and so forth), messaging apps, and online communities.

The interview with the patient and the family is an essential component in identifying patients exposed to cyberbullying and its effects, along with developing appropriate interventions. Although research on interviewing techniques for conducting the cyberbullying interview remains limited in the literature, the importance of creating a safe space, actively listening to the child, and allowing self-reflection points are critical.[43] When interviewing, one must be aware of the nuance and unique dynamics of cyberbullying and its impact on the mental health and well-being of children and adolescents.

As mentioned previously, many child victims of cyberbullying do not tell adults,[44–46] and are more likely to disclose their experiences to peers, making those relationships the more likely outlet.[47] Unfortunately, cyberbullying is also commonly neither reported nor noticed by adults.[10] Thus, it is crucial for clinicians to understand signs of cyberbullying, facilitate quality interviews, and foster safe environments.

RECOGNIZING SIGNS OF CYBERBULLYING

Understanding the signs of cyberbullying is important when incorporating it into an assessment. Many victims present psychosomatically, with physical symptoms such as recurrent abdominal pain, headaches, and difficulty with sleep.[48] In addition, growing research over the past decade has reported significant adverse physical and mental health outcomes cyberbullying has on adolescents.[9] In comparison to traditional bullying, individuals being cyberbullied may show a change in behaviors or mood, particularly when interacting with or completing the use of their device. Other signs of youth who have been victimized include anxiety, depression, or suicidal ideation. Cyberbullying perpetrators have been shown to have more mental health and external problems or low psychological well-being and quality of life.[8] When screening, it is crucial to be aware of the increased risk of cyberbullying among vulnerable youth from marginalized populations—cultural or ethnic minorities, sexual orientation minorities (LGBTQ), and youth with disabilities.[49]

CLINICAL INTERVIEW

In a clinical setting, the interviewer should begin by creating a safe environment for the child to discuss their experiences with their online use. As acts of cyberbullying commonly occur off school campuses and go unnoticed by parents, pediatric health care providers can play a crucial role in facilitating disclosure. Still, research regarding clinical setting interviews for cyberbullying remains limited. Lack of universally standardized definitions, cross-cultural differences, and self-report bias create challenges in developing standardized interviewing assessment tools to investigate cyberbullying in the clinic.[50]

Children who are being bullied may be reluctant to admit it in interviews due to fear of reliving traumatic experiences or reprisal from parents or interviewers.[47] Thus, it is helpful to allow for self-reflection and actively listen to the child rather than assume they will report it when directly asked.[43] Providers should become comfortable asking about patient's relationships with online digital platforms. In any interview, the approach to screening for cyberbullying should be sensitive, nonthreatening, and age appropriate. Begin with the use of open-ended questions around the issue and narrow focus accordingly. Some examples of questions that can be used to screen include those in **Table 1**. These questions provide a rough framework and should be adapted based on the child's age, development, and the context of the interview.

SCREENING TOOLS

The use of screening tools can also be helpful. Several screening instruments have been developed to address cyberbullying. However, few screening tools are specifically curated for clinical settings. Among the screening tools available for health care providers are the Cyberbullying and Online Aggression Survey[51,52] and the Child Adolescent Bullying Scale.[52,53] The lack of consensus in definitions, the various technology platforms, and measurement inconsistencies hinder consistent reliability and validity throughout the tools.[50]

Table 1 Examples of questions that can be used to screen children	
Question	**Purpose of Question**
What do you like to do online? What are your favorite sites or apps to use?	To open dialog about the child's online landscape without directly addressing cyberbullying
Have you ever seen or received any messages online that made you uncomfortable, scared, or upset?	To invite the child to discuss negative online interactions potentially related to cyberbullying
How do you usually handle situations online when someone says something mean or hurtful?	To gain insight into the child's coping strategies and experiences with cyberbullying
Do you ever worry about going online because of things that people might say or do?	To assess for anxiety related to online interactions, indicating possible cyberbullying
Have you or any of your friends ever been treated badly on the Internet? What happened?	To ease into the discussions of cyberbullying by starting with the child's friends' experiences
Is there anything about being online that you wish you could change?	To reveal any negative emotions tied to online activity, hinting at cyberbullying experiences
Have you ever talked to someone about bad things that happen online? Who do you feel you can talk to?	To understand the child's support network and their approach to seeking help
Sometimes kids can get picked on through their phone or computer. Has this ever happened to you?	To directly address cyberbullying in a gentle manner after establishing rapport
What do you think someone should do if they are being bullied online?	To assess the child's awareness of interventions for cyberbullying and provide an opportunity to further educate
If something happens online that makes you feel bad, what do you usually do after?	To understand the child's resilience and coping methods

Clinical case 2
Physician: "What did you like to do on your phone?"
Teen: "I used to like Instagram."
Physician: "Used to?"
Teen, sitting up straight, in a frustrated tone: "Yeah. Used to. Do you know how to make memes?"

SUPPORT

In the case example, the adolescent's recent decline in school attendance, avoidance of her device, and change in behavior upon mention of SM raise suspicion of potential cyberbullying. The complexities and nuances of cyberbullying make it difficult to detect. As such, establishing a secure, safe, and supportive environment is essential. Provide empathetic support, especially after they disclose vulnerable experiences with cyberbullying. Physicians should reassure the child or adolescent that they are not at fault and ensure they have a network of support at home and school to help them through this experience. Highlighting the widespread increase in cyberbullying can further reinforce that they are not alone in their experience.

INTERVENTIONS
School Interventions

Although cyberbullying acts are more likely to occur at home, resounding effects from the pain may carry into the school setting.[54] Research indicates school-aged children victims of cyberbullying can develop behavioral problems and adverse school outcomes.[55] As the digital world continues to integrate into the social fabric of contemporary youth, schools should understand the harms of cyberbullying and consider implementing effective strategies to protect youth.

With cyberbullying now a public health concern, there has been growing interest in preventing and addressing the issue, resulting in an increase of school-based intervention programs.[56] Cyberbullying prevention strategies may be implemented in various ways for schools. Several studies support whole-school anticyberbullying programs as the most effective.[57] Whole-school programs implement comprehensive strategies on multifaceted levels, focusing on preventing bullying and promoting online safety through school-wide culture development.[57,58] For example, the KiVa program used both targeted and universal interventions to effectively reduce the frequency of cybervictimization.[58–60] Many studies in the literature demonstrate more effective results for programs that approach the overall environment and foster a supportive school-wide culture. However, the universally focused approach is expensive and difficult to implement uniformly due to the various resources and policies across schools.[58]

School-based antibullying programs have been reported to effectively reduce cyberbullying perpetration and victimization.[55,61] Although the intervention research regarding anticyberbullying programs is scarce, the results of recent studies continue to bring promise. Gaffney indicated that anticyberbullying programs could reduce anticyberbullying perpetration by 10% to 15% and victimization by about 14%.[61] Polanin and colleagues[55] conducted a comprehensive systemic review and meta-analysis, confirming the various previous studies' findings of significantly reducing anticyberbullying perpetration and victimization, estimating a program to have a 76% and 73% reduction probability, respectively. Creating a positive school environment or reforming the environment may lead to fewer cyberbullying events among the students.[62]

Schools are leaning toward innovative ways to address cyberbullying via digital citizenship curricula, student SM contracts, and school-issued device contracts. Digital citizenship is the responsible use of technology, and schools are developing digital citizenship curricula to address cyberbullying, emphasizing ethical online behavior, empathy, and the impact of one's digital footprint. Student SM contracts encourage students to reflect on their online presence and adhere to agreed upon guidelines for respectful and safe engagement. Furthermore, school-issued device contracts explicitly outline acceptable use policies, fostering accountability and creating a framework for responsible device management. Collectively, these measures foster a safer and more considerate digital environment, empowering students to navigate the online world with integrity and awareness.

Parent Interventions

Families and parent involvement play a critical role in decreasing bullying.[63] Strong social support systems are one of the most successful prevention forms of cyberbullying.[3] Unfortunately, parents may not be aware of their child being actively cyberbullied. Hence, parental education on cyberbullying is important for prevention.[64] Educating parents about the signs of cyberbullying may broaden their understanding of the subtle severity. For example, presentations teaching the ways to respond to cyberbullying for parents have shown parents becoming more willing to engage in discussions with their children.[65,66] Common points parents should emphasize are not engaging with the perpetrator (stop, don't share, comment, or "like"), saving evidence (screenshots), and telling a trusted adult.

Parents may provide support to their youth by encouraging communication. Studies indicate that parental monitoring and open discussion are effective in cyberbullying prevention.[67] As in the clinical setting, creating a supportive space at home allows youth the opportunity to disclose events of cyberbullying. Parents can start the conversation by asking if their child has heard of cyberbullying. By engaging with their children in an open-ended, nonjudgmental manner, parents can learn about any concerning online behavior and advise of potential real-world consequences.

In some cases, parents may need teaching or training to develop appropriate methods for navigating cyberbullying situations.[68] Skills building is pivotal for cyberbullying prevention.[55,69] Skills building equips both the parent and child with techniques to implement when or after they encounter cyberbullying.[69] Common practices include promoting digital citizenship, building coping skills, and empathy training. Clinicians should advocate for parents to get involved and collaborate with the schools when concerned about cyberbullying.

Digital Interventions

Digital interventions introduce a progressive approach to combating cyberbullying. Using a variety of technologies—including videos, SM platforms, video games, and virtual reality—these interventions offer dynamic and interactive methods to educate and engage youth about cyberbullying. The programs aim to increase youth engagement and participation.

Digital programs educate youth about the signs of cyberbullying and provide them with tools to respond effectively. Beyond awareness, they provide psychoeducation, facilitate online support groups, and implement interactive activities that promote digital citizenship or teach coping skills. For example, education resources provided through the Increasing Resilience to Cyberbullying program significantly increased the likelihood of adolescents using coping skills of self-compassion.[65,70]

Recognizing that cyberbullying transcends one environment, such as the school or home, digital interventions offer accessibility spanning across various settings. SM platforms have provided a feasible outlet for remote recruiting into programs.[65,71] Furthermore, the capability of technology to foster community building presents an innovative avenue to address cyberbullying. Web-based support has been shown to be effective for individuals who have limited social connections, enhancing their access to community and resources.

Digital intervention programs creatively deliver interactive prevention content. One cyberbullying program created an interactive web-based forum, allowing students to obtain learning content, participate in discussions, and receive feedback from web-based educators.[55,72] Optimizing the immersion experience of virtual reality technology, a recent study used virtual reality to deliver interactive prevention content.[55,73] Despite the potential of digital intervention programs, challenges persist, particularly in the area of automatic detection due to nuances in web communication.[50] While digital cyberbullying programs offer innovative strategies for the prevention and intervention of cyberbullying, their efficacy requires further investigation.

AREAS LACKING SUFFICIENT RESEARCH

Cyberbullying prevention and intervention research presents several gaps and areas in need of deeper exploration. A significant challenge within this field is the absence of universally accepted definitions and measurement tools for cyberbullying. As mentioned previously, the lack of consensus in definitions and standardized measurements makes it difficult to compare findings across studies and limits the generalizability of intervention strategies.[8,50] The variability in definitions and datasets hinders the ability to achieve cross-domain generalizations.[8]

While existing literature reviews suggest some effectiveness in cyberbullying programs, the necessity for future longitudinal studies to assess these interventions' long-term effectiveness remains pressing. The current research mostly involves small sample sizes and short-term studies, requiring future longitudinal studies to evaluate the long-term effects of cyberbullying in larger samples.[8] Furthermore, there is limited research on the impact of cultural and contextual factors on cyberbullying and the effectiveness of interventions tailored to specific populations, particularly vulnerable populations of minoritized youth.

Cyberbullying's complex nature across various platforms and mediums presents a significant challenge for researchers to keep pace with rapid technological advancements and the ever-evolving digital landscape. The importance of digital literacy suggests a need for training and equipping educators with digital literacy skills for cyberbullying programs in the digital age.[50] The field of cyberbullying research is still relatively new, and these challenges highlight the importance of further longitudinal research, collaboration, and the development of effective prevention and interventions in cyberbullying.

CLINICS CARE POINTS

- Cyberbullying is a form of bullying or harassment that takes place over digital devices like computers, smartphones, and tablets.
- Though there is lack of a single definition for cyberbullying, there is consensus that cyberbullying is a significant public health issue.
- Most studies report that prevalence rates for cyberbullying range from 20% to 40%, though it is likely underreported by both victims and perpetrators.
- Minoritized youth have higher rates of victimization, with gender differences noted in certain populations.
- Cyberbullying has major negative impact on the physical and mental health of children and adolescents, including increased risk of insomnia, poor academic performance, anxiety, depression, social isolation, and even suicidal ideation.
- Most youth who are cyberbullied do not tell an adult, and it often goes unnoticed by parents.
- Clinicians can best elicit information from youth by offering a safe environment, empathetic approach, and sensitive questioning.
- Parental involvement with open communication can also encourage disclosure, particularly, if there is clinical support to parents and children with education and skill-building techniques.

- School, home, and digitally based interventions have all shown promise, but further research is needed into long-term efficacy.
- Cyberbullying is a serious public health concern that requires comprehensive approaches from multiple sources, including schools, parents, health care providers, policymakers, and communities.

REFERENCES

1. Anderson M., Faverio M., and Gottfried J., Teens, social media and technology 2023, 2023, Pew Research Center, Available at: www.pewresearch.org/internet/2023/12/11/teens-social-media-and-technology-2023/ (Accessed 5 February 2024).
2. Donegan R. Bullying and cyberbullying: history, statistics, law, prevention and analysis. Elon J Undergraduate Res Commun 2012;3:33–42.
3. Ademiluyi A, Li C, Park A. Implications and preventions of cyberbullying and social exclusion in social media: systematic review. JMIR Form Res 2022;6(1): e30286.
4. Centers for Disease Control and Prevention. Youth violence: technology and youthdprotecting your child from electronic aggression. 2014. Available at: http://www.cdc.gov/violenceprevention/pdf/ea-tipsheet-a.pdf. Accessed February 5, 2024.
5. Aboujaoude E, Savage MW, Starcevic V, et al. Cyberbullying: review of an old problem gone viral. J Adolesc Health 2015;57(1):10–8. PMID: 26095405.
6. Tokunaga RS. Following you home from school: a critical review and synthesis of research on cyberbullying victimization. Comput Hum Behav 2010;26:277–87.
7. Garett R, Lord LR, Young SD. Associations between social media and cyberbullying: a review of the literature. mHealth 2016;2:46.
8. Santre S. Cyberbullying in adolescents: a literature review. Int J Adolesc Med Health 2022;35(1):1–7.
9. Ferrara P, Ianniello F, Villani A, et al. Cyberbullying a modern form of bullying: let's talk about this health and social problem. Ital J Pediatr 2018;44:14.
10. Nixon CL. Current perspectives: the impact of cyberbullying on adolescent health. Adolesc Health Med Therapeut 2014;5:143–58.
11. Nagata JM, Trompeter N, Singh G, et al. Social epidemiology of early adolescent cyberbullying in the United States. Acad Pediatr 2022;22(8):1287–93.
12. Athanasiou K, Melegkovits E, Andrie EK, et al. Cross-national aspects of cyberbullying victimization among 14–17-year-old adolescents across seven European countries. BMC Publ Health 2018;18:800.
13. González-Cabrera J, Tourón J, Machimbarrena JM, et al. Cyberbullying in gifted students: prevalence and psychological well-being in a Spanish sample. Int J Environ Res Publ Health 2019;16:2173.
14. Lee C, Shin N. Prevalence of cyberbullying and predictors of cyberbullying perpetration among Korean adolescents. Comput Hum Behav 2017;68:352–8.
15. Safaria T. Prevalence and impact of cyberbullying in a sample of Indonesian junior high school students. The Turk Online J Educ Technol 2016;15:82–91.
16. Peled Y. Cyberbullying and its influence on academic, social, and emotional development of undergraduate students. Heliyon 2019;5(3):e01393.
17. Palasinski M. Turning assault into a "harmless prank"–teenage perspectives on happy slapping. J Interpers Violence 2013;28(9):1909–23. Epub 2013 Jan 6. PMID: 23295376.

18. Zeljka D, Vesna C, Rajkovača I, et al. Cyberbullying in early adolescence: is there a difference between urban and rural environment? Am J Biomed Sci Res 2019;1: 191–6.
19. Copp JE, Mumford EA, Taylor BG. Online sexual harassment and cyberbullying in a nationally representative sample of teens: prevalence, predictors, and consequences. J Adolesc 2021;93:202–11. Epub 2021 Nov 19. PMID: 34801812.
20. Craig W, Boniel-Nissim M, King N, et al. Social media use and cyber-bullying: a cross-national analysis of young people in 42 countries. J Adolesc Health 2020; 66(6S):S100–8. PMID: 32446603.
21. Ho SS, Chen L, Ng AP. Comparing cyberbullying perpetration on social media between primary and secondary school students. Comput Educ 2017;109:74–84.
22. Mason. Cyberbullying: a preliminary assessment for school personnel. Psychol Sch 2008;45:323–48.
23. Ybarra ML, Mitchell KJ. Youth engaging in online harassment: associations with caregiver–child relationships, Internet use, and personal characteristics. J Adolesc 2004;27:319–36.
24. Kokkinos CM, Saripanidis I. A lifestyle exposure perspective of victimization through Facebook among university students. Do individual differences matter? Comput Hum Behav 2017;74:235–45.
25. Rudert S, Reutner L, Greifeneder R, et al. Faced with exclusion: perceived facial warmth and competence influence moral judgments of social exclusion. J Exp Soc Psychol 2017;68:101–12.
26. Ybarra ML, Mitchell KJ. Prevalence and frequency of Internet harassment instigation: implications for adolescent health. J Adolesc Health 2007;41:189–95.
27. Fujikawa S, Mundy LK, Canterford L, et al. Bullying across late childhood and early adolescence: a prospective cohort of students assessed annually from grades 3 to 8. Acad Pediatr 2021;21:344–51.
28. Maoneke P, Shava F, Gamundani A, et al, ICTs use and cyberspace risks faced by adolescents in Namibia. In: Proceedings of the Second African Conference for Human Computer Interaction: Thriving Communities, December 3, 2018, Windhoek, Namibia. 2018.
29. Selkie EM, Kota R, Moreno M. Cyberbullying behaviors among female college students: witnessing, perpetration, and victimization. Coll Stud J 2016;50(2): 278–87. Medline: 28966413.
30. Soares S, Brochado S, Barros H, et al. Does cyberbullying prevalence among adolescents relate with country socioeconomic and development indicators? an ecological study of 31 countries. Violence Vict 2017;32:771–90.
31. Barlett CP, Wright MF. Longitudinal relations among cyber, physical, and relational bullying and victimization: comparing majority and minority ethnic youth. J Child Adolesc Trauma 2017;11(1):49–59.
32. Kowalski RM, Dillon E, Macbeth J, et al. Racial differences in cyberbullying from the perspective of victims and perpetrators. Am J Orthopsychiatry 2020;90: 644–52.
33. Layug A, Krishnamurthy S, McKenzie R, et al. The impacts of social media use and online racial discrimination on asian american mental health: cross-sectional survey in the United States during COVID-19. JMIR Form Res 2022; 6(9):e38589.
34. Abreu RL, Kenny MC. Cyberbullying and LGBTQ youth: a systematic literature review and recommendations for prevention and intervention. J Child Adolesc Trauma 2017;11(1):81–97. PMID: 32318140; PMCID: PMC7163911.

35. Cénat JM, Blais M, Hébert M, et al. Correlates of bullying in Quebec high school students: the vulnerability of sexual-minority youth. J Affect Disord 2015;183: 315–21.
36. Taylor C, Peter T, with McMinn TL, et al. Every class in every school: the first national climate survey on homophobia, biphobia, and transphobia in Canadian schools. Final report. Toronto: Egale Canada Human Rights Trust; 2011.
37. Kowalski RM, Toth A. Cyberbullying among youth with and without disabilities. J Child Adolesc Trauma 2017;11(1):7–15. PMID: 32318133; PMCID: PMC7158969.
38. Nicolai S, Geffner R, Stolberg R, et al. Retrospective experiences of cyberbullying and emotional outcomes on young adults who stutter. J Child Adolesc Trauma 2018;11(1):27–37. PMID: 32318135; PMCID: PMC7163874.
39. Calvete E, Orue I, Estévez A, et al. Cyberbullying in adolescents: modalities and aggressors' profile. Comput Hum Behav 2010;26:1128e35.
40. Sourander A, Brunstein klomek A, Ikonen M, et al. Psychosocial risk factors associated with cyberbullying among adolescents: a population-based study. Arch Gen Psychiatr 2010;67:720e8.
41. Van geel M, Vedder P, Tanilon J. Relationship between peer victimization, cyberbullying, and suicide in children and adolescents: a meta-analysis. JAMA Pediatr 2014;168:435e42.
42. Duong J, Bradshaw C. Associations between bullying and engaging in aggressive and suicidal behaviors among sexual minority youth: the moderating role of connectedness. J Sch Health 2014;84:636–45.
43. Mishna F, Birze A, Greenblatt A. Understanding bullying and cyberbullying through an ecological systems framework: the value of qualitative interviewing in a mixed methods approach. Int Journal of Bullying Prevention 2022;4(3):220–9.
44. Peebles E. Cyberbullying: hiding behind the screen. Paediatr Child Health 2014; 19(10):527–8.
45. Vaillancourt T, Faris R, Mishna F. Cyberbullying in children and youth: implications for health and clinical practice. Can J Psychiatr 2017;62(6):368–73.
46. Agatston PW, Kowalski R, Limber S. Students' perspectives on cyber bullying. J Adolesc Health 2007;41(6, Supplement):S59–60.
47. Cassidy W, Faucher C, Jackson M. Cyberbullying among youth: a comprehensive review of current international research and its implications and application to policy and practice. Sch Psychol Int 2013;34(6):575–612.
48. Kumar VL, Goldstein MA. Cyberbullying and adolescents. Curr Pediatr Rep 2020; 8(3):86–92.
49. Espinoza G, Wright M. Cyberbullying experiences among marginalized youth: what do we know and where do we go next? J Child Adolesc Trauma 2018; 11(1):1–5.
50. Ng ED, Chua JYX, Shorey S. The effectiveness of educational interventions on traditional bullying and cyberbullying among adolescents: a systematic review and meta-analysis. Trauma Violence Abuse 2022;23(1):132–51.
51. Patchin JW, Hinduja S. Bullies move beyond the schoolyard: a preliminary look at cyberbullying. Youth Violence Juv Justice 2006;4(2):148–69.
52. Hamburger ME, Basile KC, Vivolo AM. Measuring Bullying Victimization, Perpetration, and Bystander Experiences: A Compendium of Assessment Tools. Atlanta, GA: Centers for Disease Control and Prevention, National Center for Injury Prevention and Control; 2011. https://doi.org/10.1037/e580662011-001.
53. Hutton JS, Dudley J, Horowitz-Kraus T, et al. Associations between screen-based media use and brain white matter integrity in preschool-aged children. JAMA Pediatr 2020;174(1):e193869. https://doi.org/10.1001/jamapediatrics.2019.3869.

54. Englander EK. In: Bullying and cyberbullying: what every educator needs to know. Harvard Education Press; 2013. p. 103–24.
55. Polanin JR, Espelage DL, Grotpeter JK, et al. A systematic review and meta-analysis of interventions to decrease cyberbullying perpetration and victimization. Prev Sci 2022;23(3):439–54.
56. Myers CA, Cowie H. Cyberbullying across the lifespan of education: issues and interventions from school to university. Int J Environ Res Publ Health 2019;16(7): 1217.
57. Cantone E, Piras AP, Vellante M, et al. Interventions on bullying and cyberbullying in schools: a systematic review. Clin Pract Epidemiol Ment Health 2015;11(Suppl 1 M4):58–76.
58. Siddiqui S, Schultze-Krumbholz A. Successful and emerging cyberbullying prevention programs: a narrative review of seventeen interventions applied worldwide. Societies 2023;13(9):212.
59. Williford A, Elledge LC, Boulton AJ, et al. Effects of the KiVa antibullying program on cyberbullying and cybervictimization frequency among Finnish youth. J Clin Child Adolesc Psychol 2013;42(6):820–33.
60. Lan M, Law N, Pan Q. Effectiveness of anti-cyberbullying educational programs: a socio-ecologically grounded systematic review and meta-analysis. Comput Hum Behav 2022;130:107200. https://doi.org/10.1016/j.chb.2022.107200.
61. Gaffney H, Farrington DP, Espelage DL, et al. Are cyberbullying intervention and prevention programs effective? a systematic and meta-analytical review. Aggress Violent Behav 2019;45:134–53.
62. Acosta J, Chinman M, Ebener P, et al. Evaluation of a whole-school change intervention: findings from a two-year cluster-randomized trial of the restorative practices intervention. J Youth Adolesc 2019;48(5):876–90.
63. Hendry BP, Hellsten L ann M, McIntyre LJ, et al. Recommendations for cyberbullying prevention and intervention: a Western Canadian perspective from key stakeholders. Front Psychol 2023;14:1067484. https://doi.org/10.3389/fpsyg. 2023.1067484.
64. Hutson E, Kelly S, Militello LK. Systematic review of cyberbullying interventions for youth and parents with implications for evidence-based practice. Worldviews Evidence-Based Nurs 2018;15(1):72–9.
65. Tozzo P, Cuman O, Moratto E, et al. Family and educational strategies for cyberbullying prevention: a systematic review. IJERPH 2022;19(16):10452. https://doi. org/10.3390/ijerph191610452.
66. Roberto A, Eden J, Deiss D, et al. The short-term effects of a cyberbullying prevention intervention for parents of middle school students. IJERPH 2017;14(9): 1038.
67. Helfrich EL, Doty JL, Su YW, et al. Parental views on preventing and minimizing negative effects of cyberbullying. Child Youth Serv Rev 2020;118:105377. https://doi.org/10.1016/j.childyouth.2020.105377.
68. Lindstrom Johnson S, Waasdorp TE, Gaias LM, et al. Parental responses to bullying: understanding the role of school policies and practices. J Educ Psychol 2019;111(3):475–87.
69. Mishna F, Saini M, Solomon S. Ongoing and online: children and youth's perceptions of cyber bullying. Child Youth Serv Rev 2009;31(12):1222–8.
70. Chillemi K, Abbott JAM, Austin DW, et al. A pilot study of an online psychoeducational program on cyberbullying that aims to increase confidence and help-seeking behaviors among adolescents. Cyberpsychol, Behav Soc Netw 2020; 23(4):253–6.

71. Kutok ER, Dunsiger S, Patena JV, et al. A cyberbullying media-based prevention intervention for adolescents on instagram: pilot randomized controlled trial. JMIR Mental Health 2021;8(9):e26029. https://doi.org/10.2196/26029.
72. Menesini E, Nocentini A, Palladino BE. Empowering students against bullying and cyberbullying: evaluation of an Italian peer-ied model. Int J Conf Violence 2012;6(2):313–20.
73. Ingram KM, Espelage DL, Merrin GJ, et al. Evaluation of a virtual reality enhanced bullying prevention curriculum pilot trial. J Adolesc 2019;71:72–83.

Moving?

Make sure your subscription moves with you!

To notify us of your new address, find your **Clinics Account Number** (located on your mailing label above your name), and contact customer service at:

Email: journalscustomerservice-usa@elsevier.com

800-654-2452 (subscribers in the U.S. & Canada)
314-447-8871 (subscribers outside of the U.S. & Canada)

Fax number: 314-447-8029

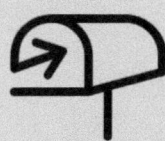

Elsevier Health Sciences Division
Subscription Customer Service
3251 Riverport Lane
Maryland Heights, MO 63043

*To ensure uninterrupted delivery of your subscription, please notify us at least 4 weeks in advance of move.

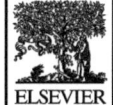